Tumors of the Parathyroid Gland

Atlas of Tumor Pathology

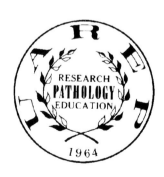

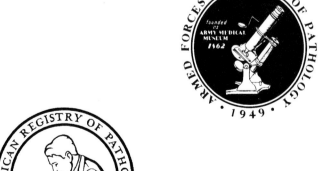

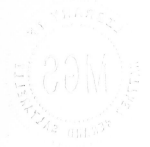

ATLAS OF TUMOR PATHOLOGY

Third Series
Fascicle 6

TUMORS OF THE
PARATHYROID GLAND

by

RONALD A. DELELLIS, M.D.
Professor, Tufts University School of Medicine
and
Senior Pathologist, New England Medical Center
Boston, Massachusetts   02111

Published by the
ARMED FORCES INSTITUTE OF PATHOLOGY
Washington, D.C.

Under the Auspices of
UNIVERSITIES ASSOCIATED FOR RESEARCH AND EDUCATION IN PATHOLOGY, INC.
Bethesda, Maryland
1993

Accepted for Publication
1991

———————————

Available from the American Registry of Pathology
Armed Forces Institute of Pathology
Washington, D.C. 20306-6000
ISSN 0160-6344
ISBN 1-881041-06-9

ATLAS OF TUMOR PATHOLOGY

EDITOR
JUAN ROSAI, M.D.
Department of Pathology
Memorial Sloan-Kettering Cancer Center
New York, New York 10021-6007

ASSOCIATE EDITOR
LESLIE H. SOBIN, M.D.
Armed Forces Institute of Pathology
Washington, D.C. 20306-6000

EDITORS' NOTE

The Atlas of Tumor Pathology has a long and distinguished history. It was first conceived at a Cancer Research Meeting held in St. Louis in September 1947 as an attempt to standardize the nomenclature of neoplastic diseases. The first series was sponsored by the National Academy of Sciences-National Research Council. The organization of this Sisyphean effort was entrusted to the Subcommittee on Oncology of the Committee on Pathology, and Dr. Arthur Purdy Stout was the first editor-in-chief. Many of the illustrations were provided by the Medical Illustration Service of the Armed Forces Institute of Pathology, the type was set by the Government Printing Office, and the final printing was done at the Armed Forces Institute of Pathology (hence the colloquial appellation "AFIP Fascicles"). The American Registry of Pathology purchased the Fascicles from the Government Printing Office and sold them virtually at cost. Over a period of 20 years, approximately 15,000 copies each of nearly 40 Fascicles were produced. The worldwide impact that these publications have had over the years has largely surpassed the original goal. They quickly became among the most influential publications on tumor pathology ever written, primarily because of their overall high quality but also because their low cost made them easily accessible to pathologists and other students of oncology the world over.

Upon completion of the first series, the National Academy of Sciences-National Research Council handed further pursuit of the project over to the newly created Universities Associated for Research and Education in Pathology (UAREP). A second series was started, generously supported by grants from the AFIP, the National Cancer Institute, and the American Cancer Society. Dr. Harlan I. Firminger became the editor-in-chief and was succeeded by Dr. William H. Hartmann. The second series Fascicles were produced as bound volumes instead of loose leaflets. They featured a more comprehensive coverage of the subjects, to the extent that the Fascicles could no longer be regarded as "atlases" but rather as monographs describing and illustrating in detail the tumors and tumor-like conditions of the various organs and systems.

Once the second series was completed, with a success that matched that of the first, UAREP and AFIP decided to embark on a third series. A new editor-in-chief and an associate editor were selected, and a distinguished editorial board was appointed. The mandate for the third series remains the same as for the previous ones, i.e., to oversee the production of an eminently practical publication with surgical pathologists as its primary audience, but also aimed at other workers in oncology. The main purposes of this series are to promote a consistent, unified, and biologically sound nomenclature; to guide the surgical pathologist in the diagnosis of the various tumors and tumor-like lesions; and to provide relevant histogenetic, pathogenetic, and clinicopathologic information on these entities. Just as the second series included data obtained from ultrastructural (and, in the more recent Fascicles, immunohistochemical) examination, the third series will, in addition, incorporate pertinent information obtained with the newer molecular biology techniques. As in the past, a continuous attempt will be made to correlate, whenever possible, the nomenclature used in the Fascicles with that proposed by the World Health Organization's International Histological Classification of Tumors. The format of the third series has been changed in order to incorporate additional items and to ensure a consistency of style throughout. This includes the dropping of the 's possessive in eponymic terms, in accordance with the WHO and the International Nomenclature of Diseases. Close cooperation between the various authors and their respective liaisons from the editorial board will be emphasized to minimize unnecessary repetition and discrepancies in the text and illustrations.

To its everlasting credit, the participation and commitment of the AFIP to this venture is even more substantial and encompassing than in previous series. It now extends to virtually all scientific, technical, and financial aspects of the production.

The task confronting the organizations and individuals involved in the third series is even more daunting than in the preceding efforts because of the ever-increasing complexity of the matter at hand. It is hoped that this combined effort—of which, needless to say, that represented by the authors is first and foremost—will result in a series worthy of its two illustrious predecessors and will be a suitable introduction to the tumor pathology of the twenty-first century.

Juan Rosai, M.D.
Leslie H. Sobin, M.D.

ACKNOWLEDGMENTS

The author wishes to express his deepest gratitude to the late Dr. Benjamin Castleman who was the author of the First Series Fascicle of Tumors of the Parathyroid Glands (1953) and to Dr. Sanford Roth who joined Dr. Castleman for the Second Series Fascicle in 1978. Both of these works have provided invaluable resources for pathologists and clinicians involved with the diagnosis and treatment of patients with hyperparathyroidism. The task of compiling this Third Series Fascicle of Tumors of the Parathyroid Glands has been made considerably easier by having both of these volumes as points of reference.

The author is also grateful to a number of individuals who contributed directly or indirectly to the preparation of this volume. Dr. Juan Rosai, the Editor-in-Chief of the Third Series, not only shared interesting case material but also offered helpful suggestions throughout all phases of the preparation of the text. Special thanks are also due to the anonymous reviewers who provided invaluable critiques.

The author also wishes to thank Dr. James Oertel, former Chief of the Endocrinology Branch, Armed Forces Institute of Pathology, for making available his extensive collection of cases of parathyroid carcinoma. Drs. Robert Erlandson (Department of Pathology, Memorial Sloan-Kettering Cancer Center, NY) and Salvatore Allegra (Department of Pathology, St. Joseph's Hospital, Providence, RI) graciously shared their entire collections of electron micrographs of diseases of the parathyroid glands.

The staff and residents from the Departments of Pathology and Surgery, New England Medical Center Hospital and Tufts University School of Medicine, provided a continual source of encouragement and support. Special thanks are due to Gerry Parker, who prepared most of the photographic material, and to Lisa Hansbury for her expert and exceptionally patient secretarial assistance.

Ronald A. DeLellis, M.D.

TUMORS OF THE PARATHYROID GLAND

Contents

TUMORS OF THE PARATHYROID GLANDS

INTRODUCTION

Ivar Sandström (1852-1889) is generally credited with the first comprehensive description of the parathyroid glands in humans in 1880, although these glands were originally recognized by Virchow seventeen years earlier (6,32). Sandström chose the name *glandulae parathyreoideae* to indicate the characteristic location of the four small glands next to the thyroid. The physiologic significance of the parathyroid glands, however, was unknown until experimental studies revealed that their removal resulted in tetany and that the tetany was associated with low levels of serum calcium (6). The observation that the administration of parathyroid gland extract was capable of reversing hypocalcemia in parathyroidectomized animals led to the discovery and ultimate characterization of parathyroid hormone (6).

THE NORMAL PARATHYROID GLAND

EMBRYOLOGY

Detailed accounts of the development of the parathyroid glands are provided by Gilmour (15), Norris (29), and Weller (35). A brief review of the embryology, however, is necessary for an understanding of the variations in the distribution of these glands in normal individuals (9,10).

The parathyroid glands are derived from the third and fourth branchial pouches. They are first recognizable in the 8 to 9 mm embryo (5 to 6 weeks of development) as localized thickenings of the antero-dorsal branchial pouch epithelium (10). The inferior parathyroid glands, together with the thymus, are derived from the third pouch and for that reason are also referred to as parathyroid III.

The derivatives of the third pouch show a complex pattern of migration and descent before they attain their final position caudad to the derivatives of the fourth pouch. Parathyroid III separates from the thymus at the 18 mm stage of development; at this stage it is at the level of the lower pole of the thyroid. Failure of parathyroid III to separate from the thymus results in the appearance of this gland in the lower neck (within the thymic tongue), anterior mediastinum, or even the posterior mediastinum. Early separation of parathyroid III from the thymus may result in the final position of this gland cephalad to the thyroid and parathyroid IV.

Thus, parathyroid III or its remnants may be found along the entire course of migration of the third pouch derivatives from the angle of the jaw to the pericardium (26).

Parathyroid IV develops from the fourth branchial pouch together with the ultimobranchial body (15,29,35). It then separates from the ultimobranchial body and assumes its final position as the upper gland. The position of parathyroid IV is close to the point where the inferior thyroid artery crosses the recurrent laryngeal nerve at the cricothyroid junction. Parathyroid IV tends to be more constant in position than parathyroid III.

In the fetus, the parathyroids are recognizable as well-vascularized, localized collections of vacuolated chief cells which are separated from the surrounding soft tissue by a thin connective tissue capsule (fig. 1).

ANATOMY

Gross Anatomy

The parathyroid glands are flattened, ovoid, or bean-shaped structures, with occasional glands having an elongated, bilobed, or multilobed configuration. They generally measure 4 to 6 mm in length, 2 to 4 mm in width, and 1 to 2 mm in thickness. Ghandur-Mnaymneh and co-workers (14) report a 95 percent upper limit for gland

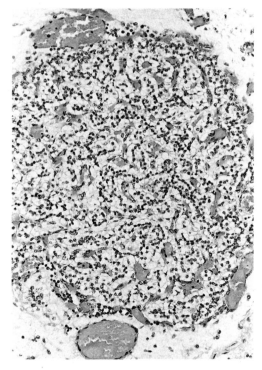

Figure 1
FETAL PARATHYROID (22 WEEKS' GESTATION)
The gland at this stage consists of vacuolated chief cells.

length of 9 mm for healthy subjects and of 10 mm for hospitalized subjects. The lower glands may be somewhat larger than the upper glands.

The average combined weight of the glands is 120 ± 3.5 mg for males and 142 ± 5.2 mg for females (18,19), with a maximum total glandular weight of 208 mg (95 percent upper limit) (19,20). In a series of 368 autopsy cases, Grimelius and co-workers (19,20) found a mean glandular weight of 32 mg, and a maximum gland weight of 59 mg (95 percent upper limit of gland weight). Ghandur-Mnaymneh and co-workers (14) reported that gland weights were greater in hospitalized patients (mean 46.2 mg) than in patients who died suddenly (39.5 mg) and a 95 percent upper limit of gland weight of 73.1 mg for healthy white subjects and 91.6 mg for healthy black subjects. Most pathologists, however, consider gland weights in excess of 40 mg abnormal.

The importance of determining parenchymal weight using planimetry or density gradients has been stressed by several groups for assessment of normal and abnormal functional states (fig. 2) (2–4,20). The mean parenchymal weight of a single gland is 22 mg with a 95 percent upper

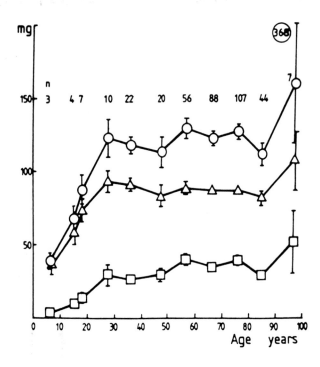

Figure 2
NORMAL PARATHYROID
WEIGHTS
The total glandular weight (opened circle), total parenchymal cell weight (opened triangle), and total fat tissue weight (opened square) are shown in relation to patient age. Mean values ± SEM. N = number of cases in each age group. The number in the upper right circle is the total number of cases. (From Grimelius L, Akerström G, Johansson H, Bergström R. Anatomy and histopathology of human parathyroid glands. Pathol Annu 1981;16(Pt 2):1–20.)

limit of 39 mg (19). The mean parenchymal weight in adults represents 74 percent of the total glandular weight; the amount of stromal adipose tissue is dependent to some extent on constitutional factors, including the amount of body fat. In individuals less than 18 years of age, parenchymal weights and total glandular weights are almost identical (figs. 2, 3). After age 18, the amount of stromal adipose tissue increases to 10 to 30 percent of the glandular volume, but the parenchymal weight remains more or less constant throughout life (figs. 2–5). There may be considerable variation in the cellularity of different glands in the same individual (5).

The color of the normal gland is red-brown when there is a high parenchymal cell to stromal fat ratio and yellow-brown when the glands contain abundant stromal fat (16). Most normal adults (84 percent) have four parathyroid glands. Akerström and co-workers (4) report 13 percent of normal individuals have more than four glands while 3 percent have only three. The lower combined total parathyroid weights in those cases in which only three glands were found suggests that a fourth parathyroid may have been missed during the dissection.

The superior pair of parathyroids (IV) is found most commonly within a circumscribed area at a distance of approximately 1 cm above the intersection of the recurrent laryngeal nerve and the inferior thyroid artery (fig. 6) (34). Generally, the glands are present in the connective tissue which binds the posterior edge of the thyroid to the pharynx. Occasionally, glands may be present within the thyroid capsule, and rarely, within the substance of the thyroid (0.2 percent) (9,10). In exceptional instances, the superior parathyroids may be found in the retropharyngeal or retroesophageal space (4).

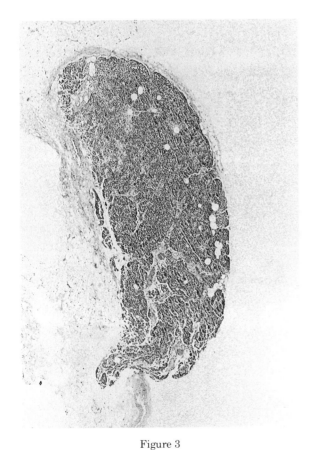

Figure 3
NORMAL PARATHYROID GLAND
In this parathyroid gland from a 12-year-old male a few stromal fat cells are present.

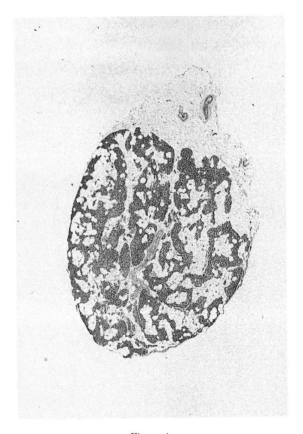

Figure 4
NORMAL ADULT PARATHYROID
In this parathyroid gland from a 40-year-old male there is a normal ratio of parenchymal cells to fat cells.

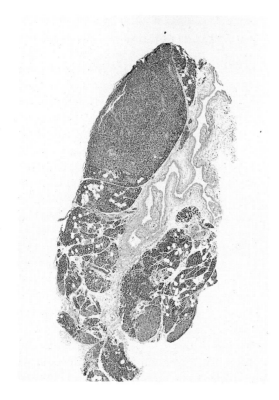

Figure 5
NORMAL ADULT PARATHYROID
In this parathyroid from a 65-year-old male a large oncocytic nodule is present in the upper pole of the gland. Several smaller oncocytic nodules are present in the lower portion of the gland. The serum calcium and phosphorus levels were normal.

DISTRIBUTION OF PARATHYROID GLANDS

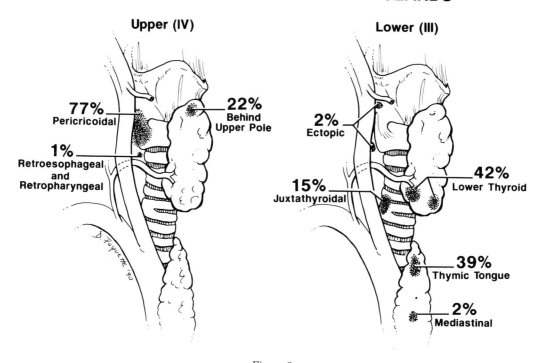

Figure 6
DISTRIBUTION OF PARATHYROID GLANDS
The thyroid lobes have been reflected anteriorly. (Adapted from Wang C. The anatomic basis of parathyroid surgery. Ann Surg 1976;183:271–5.)

The inferior parathyroids (III) are much more variable in their distribution than are the superior glands (IV), as might be anticipated from their embryologic development (33). In a study by Akerström (4), 61 percent of the inferior glands were found inferior, posterior, or lateral to the lower pole of the thyroid and 17 percent were present high up on the anterior aspect of the thyroid lobe. Other common sites of the inferior glands included the thyrothymic ligament and the cervical portion of the thymus. Inferior glands were located in the lower thymus in 2 percent of cases, and in the anterior mediastinum below the thymus in 0.2 percent of cases. In this series, 2.8 percent of inferior glands (identifiable as inferior glands by the presence of surrounding thymus) were found above the point of intersection of the recurrent laryngeal nerve and the inferior thyroid artery. A small number of inferior glands were also located within the posterior mediastinum. Despite variations in their positions within the neck, the distribution of the parathyroids tends to be bilaterally symmetrical.

The arterial supply of the glands is derived from branches of the superior thyroid artery (upper or parathyroid IV) and the inferior thyroid artery (lower or parathyroid III). However, there may be considerable variability in the arterial supplies of the glands, depending on their anatomic locations in the neck (10). Venous drainage of the upper glands occurs via the superior or lateral thyroid vein, while drainage of the lower glands occurs via the lateral or inferior thyroid vein. Lymphatic drainage originates from a subcapsular plexus into the superior deep cervical, pretracheal, paratracheal, retropharyngeal, and inferior deep cervical nodes.

True supernumerary glands, defined as being located apart from the other four glands and weighing more than 5 mg, are identifiable in approximately 5 percent of individuals. Most patients with true supernumerary parathyroids have 5 glands, a few have 6 glands, and a very few have up to 11 glands. In most patients with more than 4 glands, the supernumerary glands are either rudimentary (less than 5 mg) or split (divided) (4,16). True supernumerary glands are found most commonly in the thymus or in relation to the thyrothymic ligament (3). Supernumerary glands have also been found in the submucosa of the esophagus and the hypopharynx (26).

Lack and co-workers (26) found supernumerary or ectopic parathyroid tissue in 6 percent of vagus nerves of 32 children up to 1 year of age. The collections of parathyroid tissue ranged from 162 to 360 µm in diameter. Rarely, normal parathyroid tissue may be found in extremely unusual anatomic sites, such as the vaginal wall (25).

Agenesis of the parathyroid glands is rare. In patients with the DiGeorge syndrome, there is complete or partial absence of the third and fourth pharyngeal pouch complexes, including the thymus, parathyroid glands, and C cells (8). Affected individuals also show evidence of facial, skeletal, and cardiovascular abnormalities.

Microscopic Anatomy

The parathyroids are richly vascularized and are demarcated from the surrounding structures of the neck by a thin connective tissue capsule (see figs. 3–5) (1,17). Blood vessels enter and leave the gland via fibrous trabecula which extend from the capsule. Although the parathyroids are innervated, the role of neural control of physiological function of the glands is unknown.

Occasional small collections or nests of chief cells may be seen external to the gland capsules within the surrounding soft tissues of the neck or mediastinum. In patients with primary and secondary chief cell hyperplasia, parathyroid nests and supernumerary glands may also become hyperplastic, and this finding has been referred to as *parathyromatosis* (30).

The parenchymal elements of the parathyroid include chief cells, varying numbers of oncocytic cells, and transitional oncocytic cells (1,10). The parenchymal cells are often arranged in a lobular pattern, particularly in adults (figs. 5, 7).

Chief cells are generally polyhedral and measure 8 to 10 µm in diameter (fig. 8) (1). The nuclei are round, centrally positioned, and have coarse chromatin with well-defined nuclear membranes. Because of the density of their chromatin, the nuclei often appear pyknotic, particularly in thick sections. Mitoses are almost never seen in normal adult parathyroids.

The cytoplasm of chief cells in well-fixed samples is generally eosinophilic to amphophilic. In formalin-fixed tissues, the cytoplasm often has a clear or somewhat vacuolated appearance (fig. 8). The cells are typically well glycogenated and

5

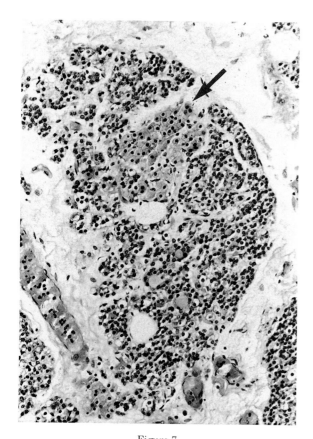

Figure 7
NORMAL ADULT PARATHYROID
Lobule of parathyroid contains chief cells and a small cluster of oncocytic cells (arrow). Scattered glandular structures contain colloid.

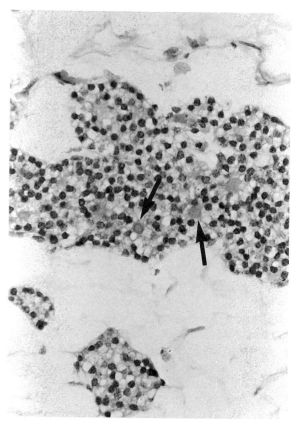

Figure 8
NORMAL ADULT PARATHYROID
Many chief cells contain a large single cytoplasmic vacuole. Glandular structures contain colloid (arrow).

contain variable amounts of neutral lipid in the form of 2 to 3 sudanophilic fat droplets per cell (pl. I–A). Fat droplets are present in approximately 80 percent of the chief cells in resting adult glands and in 30 to 40 percent of chief cells in glands from infants and children (1).

Chief cells with clear cytoplasm should be distinguished from the water-clear cells (wasserhelle cells) which are found in clear cell hyperplasia. The water-clear cells contain multiple cytoplasmic vacuoles best demonstrated in 1-μm-thick plastic embedded sections.

In glands with little stromal fat, chief cells are arranged in solid sheets (see fig. 3). With increasing fat content, the chief cells tend to form branching and anastomosing cords (see fig. 4) (10,19). Chief cells may also form small acinar or glandular structures and occasional follicles con-

taining an eosinophilic PAS-positive material resembling colloid may be seen (figs. 7, 8). The colloid, in some instances, is also strongly congophilic and shows green birefringence typical of amyloid (10,19).

The oncocytic cells measure 12 to 20 μm in diameter and are characterized by the presence of deeply eosinophilic cytoplasmic granules (fig. 9; pl. I–B). The nucleus is somewhat larger than that of the chief cell (10,19). Oncocytic cells are rich in oxidative enzymes and contain abundant mitochondria. They typically appear at puberty and increase in number with age, characteristically forming clusters and nodules (see fig. 5). Large oncocytic nodules may be impossible to distinguish from oncocytic adenomas. Transitional oncocytic cells are smaller and less eosinophilic than mature oncocytic cells.

PLATE I

NORMAL ADULT PARATHYROID

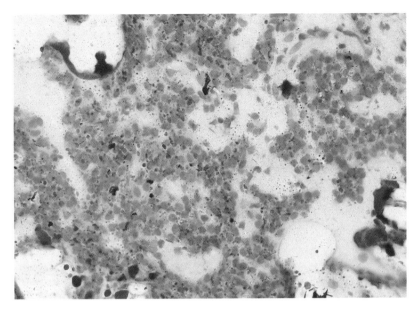

A. Neutral lipid deposits are present both within the stromal fat cells and within the parenchymal cells (frozen section, oil red O).

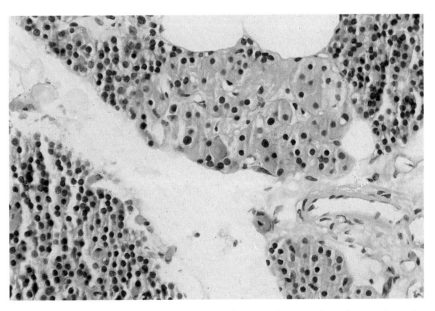

B. The oncocytes have granular eosinophilic cytoplasm and are larger than the surrounding chief cells.

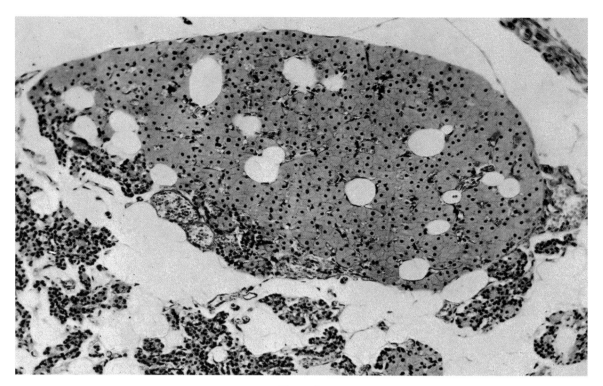

Figure 9
ONCOCYTIC NODULE
In this oncocytic nodule from the parathyroid of an elderly individual, the oncocytic cells have hyperchromatic central nuclei and abundant granular cytoplasm. Fat cells are present within the nodule. (Fig. 4 from Fascicle 15, First Series.)

The stromal compartment of the parathyroid includes mature fat cells, blood vessels, and varying amounts of connective tissue (11,12). The amount of stromal connective tissue increases with the age of the individual. Generally, the parathyroid glands of infants and children contain little fibrous tissue, while those of adults contain more abundant fibrous tissue, which tends to accentuate the lobular appearance of the glands (1).

Evaluation of the proportions of stromal fat and parenchymal elements has been considered important for correlation of gland morphology with normal and abnormal functional states. Until adolescence, the number of stromal fat cells is minimal although obese children tend to have more stromal fat than do normal or lean children. The number of stromal fat cells increases until the ages of 25 to 30; in older individuals the amount of stromal fat is determined primarily by constitutional factors.

Although earlier studies indicated that adult parathyroid glands contained approximately 50 percent stromal fat, more recent analyses employing point counting morphometry show that the amount of stromal fat is considerably lower. In a study of parathyroid glands obtained at autopsy, two thirds of the glands had less than 20 percent stromal fat while only 9 percent had more than 40 percent stromal fat (11). In a study of normal parathyroids reported by Dufour and Wilkerson (12), the average parathyroid stromal fat content was 17 percent. Only one patient from this series had more than 50 percent stromal fat, and almost one third had less than 10 percent (12).

Stromal fat is often irregularly distributed within the glands; the polar regions tend to be richer in stromal fat than the more central regions (4,19). Biopsies from the poles may, therefore, give spuriously high stromal fat to parenchymal cell ratios. The validity of estimating

PLATE II

NORMAL ADULT PARATHYROID

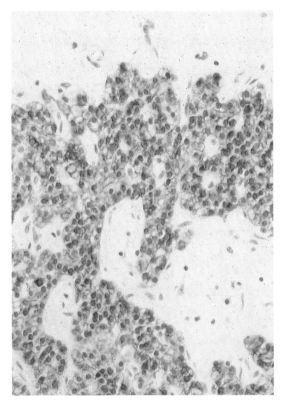

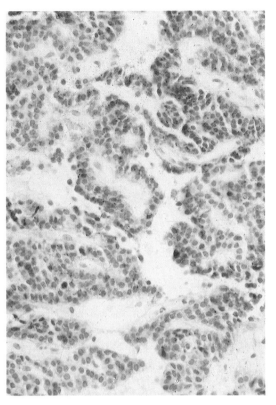

A. Paraffin section stained for low molecular weight keratins, avidin biotin peroxidase technique. Each cell contains keratin in periphery of cytoplasm.

B. Paraffin section stained for parathyroid hormone, avidin biotin peroxidase technique. Faint staining is present in many chief cells.

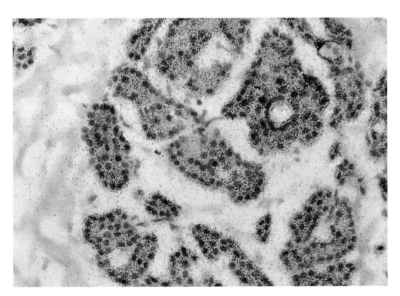

C. Autoradiograph, in situ hybridization using a 35-S–labeled antisense RNA probe for pre-pro-parathyroid hormone mRNA. All of the parathyroid cells are intensely labeled. (Courtesy of Dr. Hubert J. Wolfe, Boston, MA.)

stromal fat to parenchymal cell ratios from a few sections of intact glands and from surgical biopsies is questionable. Such biopsies are of value only in identifying tissue type.

An objective estimate of the ratio of parenchymal cells to stromal fat can be obtained by density measurements. The results of studies using this approach indicate that there is an almost linear relationship between parenchymal cell content and glandular density (20). Such measurements, performed with an isosmotic gradient medium, such as Percoll, can then be used in conjunction with measurements of total gland weight in order to derive parenchymal cell weight (4,20).

HISTOCHEMISTRY AND IMMUNOHISTOCHEMISTRY

Glycogen is present in the vast majority of chief cells, as demonstrated by the periodic acid–Schiff stain. The glycogen content of oxyphil cells is less than that of chief cells. Neutral lipid droplets are demonstrable in most normal chief cells using oil red O or Sudan IV (see pl. I–A), while oncocytes do not contain significant amounts of neutral lipid (1).

Immunohistochemical studies (27) have demonstrated that the parathyroid chief cells contain cytokeratins 8 (52kD), 18 (45kD), and 19 (40kD) (pl. II–A). Oncocytic cells contain cytokeratins of identical molecular weights although the intensity of staining is less than that of chief cells. Vimentin is present within stromal and vascular endothelial cells, but absent from the parenchymal cells. Neurofilament proteins and neuron-specific enolase have been reported in occasional parenchymal cells of parathyroid adenomas but not in normal parathyroids (27,38).

The localization of parathyroid hormone in normal and adenomatous parathyroid tissue has proven to be difficult, partly because of the relatively low rates of hormone storage within individual chief cells. Moreover, some of the antibodies used in immunohistochemical staining formats may react only with the amino terminal, midportion, or the carboxy terminal portions of the hormone (pl. II–B).

With antibodies to bovine parathyroid hormone, positive staining has been observed within the chief cells and to a lesser extent within oncocytic cells (13,21,37). Ultrastructural immunocytochemical studies have demonstrated that the positive staining is confined to the secretory granules.

An alternative approach to the demonstration of parathyroid hormone is the use of molecular probes for parathyroid hormone messenger RNA. Stork and co-workers (33) utilized S-35–labeled antisense RNA probes for pre–pro-parathyroid hormone messenger RNA both in frozen and paraffin-embedded sections (pl. II–C). In normal parathyroids, chief cells and transitional oncocytic cells show a relatively high steady state expression of parathyroid messenger RNA, while oncocytic cells show a low hybridization signal. Similar results were reported by Kendall and co-workers (24) using digoxigenin-labeled probes. The use of in situ hybridization appears to be more useful than immunohistochemistry for demonstrating the ability of cells to produce parathyroid hormone.

Juhlin and co-workers (22,23) generated monoclonal antibodies to a receptor on parathyroid cells involved in the sensing and gating of calcium. These antibodies react with the cell surface of chief cells and the proximal tubule cells of the kidney. Immunohistochemical studies have revealed intense staining of the parenchymal cells of normal and suppressed glands, while adenomas and cases of hyperplasia exhibit reduced staining. Metastases of two parathyroid carcinomas revealed intense staining. These antibodies may, therefore, be valuable reagents for the analysis of parathyroid biopsies.

Parathyroid secretory protein has also been demonstrated within the parathyroid with immunohistochemical methods. Ultrastructural studies have revealed that this protein is co-localized with parathyroid hormone within secretory granules. Parathyroid secretory protein is closely related to chromogranin A, and antibodies to chromogranin A show positive but weak reactions within parathyroid chief cells (1,36).

The oxidative enzymes of parathyroid cells have also been studied both by histochemical and immunohistochemical methods. Bedetti and co-workers (7) demonstrated cytochrome C oxidase immunoreactivity, particularly in oncocytic cells, while transitional oncocytic cells showed intermediate levels of staining and chief cells stained weakly or negatively.

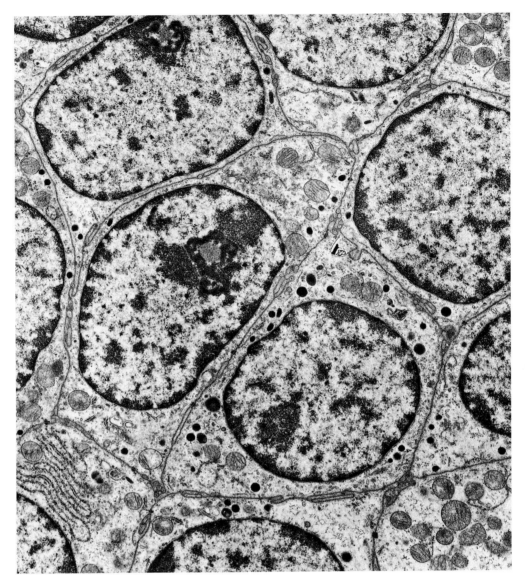

Figure 10
ELECTRON MICROGRAPH OF NORMAL PARATHYROID
Occasional dense core secretory granules are evident (X12,700).

ULTRASTRUCTURE

The ultrastructural characteristics of the normal parathyroid gland have been studied by several groups (28,31). The parenchymal cells of the gland are arranged in varying sized cords and nests which are separated from the interstitial space by a well-formed basal lamina. The surrounding capillaries are lined by endothelial cells with fenestrations similar to those seen in other endocrine glands (1).

Chief cells in their resting phases generally have relatively straight plasma membranes, and are connected to adjacent cells via desmosomal attachments (fig. 10). Increased functional activity is associated with greater tortuosity of the plasma membranes. Chief cells contain moderate numbers of mitochondria which are distributed randomly throughout the cytoplasm (figs. 10, 11).

Glycogen deposits may be prominent in some cells. The endoplasmic reticulum is most often located in a perinuclear position, but occasional

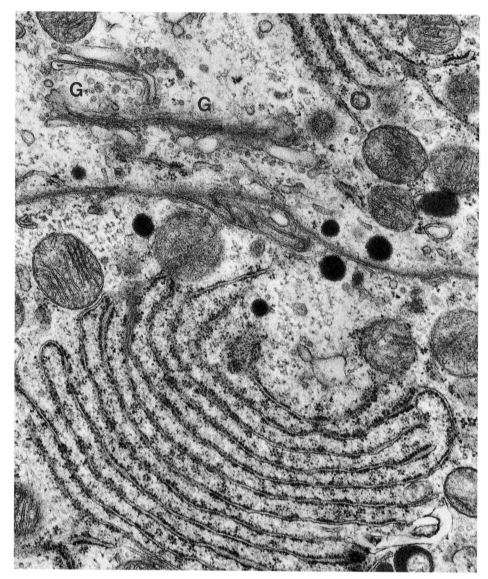

Figure 11
ELECTRON MICROGRAPH OF
NORMAL PARATHYROID
The upper cell shows Golgi (G) saccules and vesicles, some of which contain moderately electron dense material. The lower cell shows prominent stacks of granular endoplasmic reticulum. Electron dense secretory granules are present in both cells (X39,000).

cisternae may also be located peripherally. The Golgi regions are characterized by the presence of widened saccules and small empty-appearing vesicles.

The prosecretory granules measure up to 0.2 mm in diameter and are generally round in outline. These granules are recognized by the presence of centrally located, moderately electron dense cores which are separated from their limiting membranes by a lucent space. Prosecretory granules are most often located adjacent to the Golgi regions or adjacent to the plasma membranes.

Mature secretory granules contain material which is more dense than that seen in prosecretory granules and which generally fills the space delineated by the surrounding granule membrane (see figs. 10, 11). Most secretory granules are round and measure up to 0.3 μm in diameter. Some, however, have an ovoid or dumbbell configuration which sometimes makes their differentiation from lysosomes difficult. Lysosomes are generally the same size as secretory granules, but they tend to be more pleomorphic with round, ovoid, or rod-like configurations. In contrast to secretory granules, lysosomes are rich in acid phosphatase.

In the resting phase, chief cells contain abundant glycogen and lipids (1,10,31). The solitary lipid droplets measure up to 1 μm in diameter, while complex or conglomerate lipid droplets may measure up to 5 μm. Granular endoplasmic reticulum and ribosomes are dispersed throughout the cytoplasm, and the cells contain relatively few secretory and prosecretory granules.

Chief cells in an active synthetic phase are somewhat smaller than resting chief cells and contain decreased amounts of glycogen and lipid. The granular endoplasmic reticulum is present in the form of multiple parallel stalks. In the packaging phase of the secretory cycle the cells are small but show a high degree of plasma membrane tortuosity. The Golgi region is prominently developed with numerous vesicles and prosecretory granules. In the secretory phase, the cells increase in size and secretory granules move towards the plasma membranes. With involution, the cells further enlarge with the accumulation of lipid and glycogen, while the plasma membranes become relatively straight.

Oncocytic cells are characterized by the presence of numerous mitochondria that fill the cytoplasm and that are generally larger than those seen in chief cells (fig. 12). While most mitochondria are ovoid, some may be elongated or dumbbell shaped. The endoplasmic reticulum is less abundant than in chief cells and the Golgi regions tend to be considerably smaller. Both prosecretory and secretory granules are present in

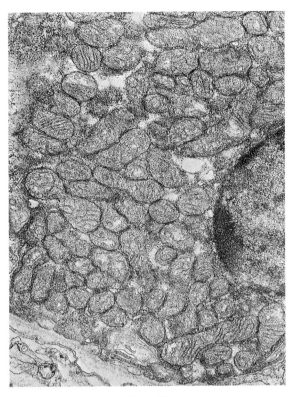

Figure 12
ELECTRON MICROGRAPH OF
NORMAL PARATHYROID
This oncocytic cell is filled with mitochondria. (Fig. 15 from Fascicle 14, Second Series.)

smaller numbers than in chief cells as are lipid inclusions.

Transitional oncocytic cells contain fewer mitochondria than oncocytic cells but more mitochondria than chief cells. Both the endoplasmic reticulum and Golgi regions are smaller than in oncocytic cells. Vesicles, prosecretory granules, and mature secretory granules are fewer in transitional oncocytic cells than in chief cells, but their relative numbers are approximately the same.

REFERENCES

1. Abu-Jawdeh GM, Roth SI. Parathyroid glands. In: Sternberg SS, ed. Histology for pathologists. New York: Raven Press, 1992:311–20.

2. Akerström G, Grimelius L, Johansson H, Lundqvist H, Pertoft H, Bergström R. The parenchymal cell mass in normal human parathyroid glands. Acta Pathol Microbiol Immunol Scand [A] 1981;89:367–75.

3. _____, Grimelius L, Johansson H, Pertroft H, Lundqvist H. Estimation of the parathyroid parenchymal cell mass by density gradients. Am J Pathol 1980;99: 685–94.

4. _____, Malmaeus J, Bergström R. Surgical anatomy of human parathyroid glands. Surgery 1984;95:14–21.

5. _____, Rudberg C, Grimelius L, et al. Histologic parathyroid abnormalities in an autopsy series. Hum Pathol 1986;17:520–7.

6. Allbright F. A page out of the history of hyperparathyroidism. J Clin Endocrinol Metab 1948;8:637–57.

7. Bedetti CD. Immunocytochemical demonstration of cytochrome C oxidase with an immunoperoxidase method: A specific stain for mitochondria in formalin-fixed and paraffin-embedded tissues. J Histochem Cytochem 1985;33:446–52.

8. Burke BA, Johnson D, Gilbert EF, et al. Thyrocalcitonin containing cells in the DiGeorge anomaly. Hum Pathol 1987;18:355–60.

9. Castleman B. Tumors of the parathyroid glands. Atlas of Tumor Pathology. Sect. IV, Fascicle 15. Washington, D.C.: Armed Forces Institute of Pathology, 1952.

10. _____, Roth SI. Tumors of the parathyroid glands. Atlas of Tumor Pathology, 2nd Series, Fascicle 14. Washington, D.C.: Armed Forces Institute of Pathology, 1978, 1–94.

11. Dekker A, Dunsford HA, Geyer SJ. The normal parathyroid gland at autopsy: the significance of stromal fat in adult patients. J Pathol 1979;128:127–32.

12. Dufour DR, Wilkerson SY. The normal parathyroid revisited: percentage of stromal fat. Hum Pathol 1982;13:717–21.

13. Futrell JM, Roth SI, Su SP, Habenar JF, Segre GV, Potts JT Jr. Immunocytochemical localization of parathyroid hormone in bovine parathyroid glands and human parathyroid adenomas. Am J Pathol 1979;94:615–22.

14. Ghandur-Mnaymneh L, Cassady J, Hajianpour MA, Paz J, Reiss E. The parathyroid gland in health and disease. Am J Pathol 1986;125:292–9.

15. Gilmour JR. The embryology of the parathyroid glands, the thymus and certain associated rudiments. J Pathol 1937;45:507–22.

16. _____. The gross anatomy of the parathyroid glands. J Pathol 1938;46:133–49.

17. _____. The normal histology of the parathyroid glands. J Pathol 1939;48:187–222.

18. _____, Martin WJ. The weight of the parathyroid glands. J Pathol 1937;44:431–62.

19. Grimelius L, Åkerström G, Johansson H, Juhlin C, Rastad J. The parathyroid glands. In: Kovacs K, Asa S, eds. Functional endocrine pathology, Vol. 1. Boston: Blackwell Scientific, 1990:375–95.

20. _____, Akerström G, Johansson H, Bergström R. Anatomy and histopathology of human parathyroid glands. Pathol Annu 1981;16(Pt 2):1–24.

21. Hargis GK, Yakulis VJ, Williams GA, White AA. Cytological detection of parathyroid hormone by immunofluorescence. Proc Soc Exp Biol Med 1964;117:836–9.

22. Juhlin C, Akerström G, Klareskog L, et al. Monoclonal antiparathyroid antibodies revealing defect expression of a calcium receptor mechanism in hyperparathyroidism. World J Surg 1988;12:552–8.

23. _____, Holmdahl R, Johansson H, Rastad J, Akerström G, Klareskog L. Monoclonal antibodies with exclusive reactivity against parathyroid cells and tubule cells of the kidney. Proc Natl Acad Sci USA 1987;84:2990–4.

24. Kendall CH, Roberts PA, Pringle JH, Lauder I. The expression of parathyroid hormone messenger RNA in normal and abnormal parathyroid tissue. J Pathol 1991;165:111–8.

25. Kurman RJ, Prabha AC. Thyroid and parathyroid glands in the vaginal wall: Report of a case. Am J Clin Pathol 1973;59:503–7.

26. Lack EE, Delay S, Linnoila RI. Ectopic parathyroid tissue within the vagus nerve: incidence and possible clinical significance. Arch Pathol Lab Med 1988;112:304–6.

27. Miettinen M, Clark R, Lehto VP, Virtanen I, Damjanov I. Intermediate-filament proteins in parathyroid glands and parathyroid adenomas. Arch Pathol Lab Med 1985; 109:986–9.

28. Nilsson O. Studies on the ultrastructure of the human parathyroid glands in various pathological conditions. Acta Pathol Microbiol Immunol Scand [A] 1977;263 (Suppl):1–88.

29. Norris EH. The parathyroid glands and the lateral thyroid in man: their morphogenesis, histogenesis, topographic anatomy and prenatal growth. Contrib Embryol 1937;26:247–94.

30. Reddick RL, Costa JC, Marx SJ. Parathyroid hyperplasia and parathyromatosis [Letter]. Lancet 1977;1:549.

31. Roth SI, Capen CC. Ultrastructural and functional correlations of the parathyroid gland. Int Rev Exp Pathol 1974;13:161–221.

32. Sandstrom IV. On a new gland in man and several mammals—glandulae parathyroidae. Upsala Lakareforenings Forh (Proc Ups Soc Phys) 1879-1880;15:441–71.

33. Stork PJ, Herteaux C, Frazier R, Kronenberg H, Wolfe HJ. Expression and distribution of parathyroid hormone and parathyroid hormone messenger RNA in pathological conditions of the parathyroid. Lab Invest 1989;60:92A.

34. Wang C. The anatomic basis of parathyroid surgery. Ann Surg 1976;183:271–5.

35. Weller GL Jr. Development of the thyroid, parathyroid and thymus glands in man. Contrib Embryol 1933; 141:93–139.

36. Wilson BS, Lloyd RV. Detection of chromogranin in neuroendocrine cells with a monoclonal antibody. Am J Pathol 1984;115:458–68.

37. Winkler B, Gooding GA, Montgomery CK, et al. Immunoperoxidase confirmation of parathyroid origin of ultrasound-guided fine needle aspirates of the parathyroid glands. Acta Cytol 1987;31:40–4.

38. Zabel M, Dietel M. S-100 protein and neuron-specific enolase in parathyroid glands and C-cells of the thyroid. Histochemistry 1987;86:389–92.

PHYSIOLOGY

NORMAL PHYSIOLOGY

PARATHYROID HORMONE BIOSYNTHESIS

Parathyroid hormone is an 84 amino acid peptide (molecular weight 9,500) encoded by a gene on the short arm of chromosome 11 (25). The hormone is synthesized within the cytoplasm of the chief cell, and to a lesser extent within the oncocytes, as a 115 amino acid–containing precursor, pre–pro-parathyroid hormone. The precursor enters the endoplasmic reticulum where the 25 amino acid–containing N-terminal portion of the molecule is removed. The resultant intermediary protein, pro-parathyroid hormone, is then transported to the Golgi region where cleavage of the hexapeptide-containing N-terminal segment of the molecule occurs. In this manner, pro-parathyroid hormone is converted to parathyroid hormone. From the Golgi region, parathyroid hormone is transported to secretory granules where it is stored, together with parathyroid secretory protein, prior to release into the circulation (3,4,25). Subsequent events in the liver and other sites convert parathyroid hormone to C-terminal and N-terminal fragments which can be measured by radioimmunoassay. The half-life of the biologically active N-terminal fragment of the hormone is considerably shorter than that of the inactive C-terminal fragment.

CALCIUM HOMEOSTASIS

Calcium and phosphorus levels are controlled by the actions of three major hormones: parathyroid hormone, calcitriol (1,25[OH]$_2$D$_3$), and calcitonin (25). These hormones regulate mineral homeostasis by their actions on bone, kidney, and intestine (1a).

Under normal conditions, the concentration of calcium in the serum ranges from 9 to 10.5 mg/dl (2.2 to 2.6 mmol/l). Calcium is distributed in three major fractions in the extracellular fluid. Forty-six percent is bound to protein, 48 percent is present as ionized calcium (12), and the remainder is associated with diffusible ion complexes.

Ionized calcium is the most important regulator of the biosynthesis and secretion of parathyroid hormone (1a). Increased levels of ionized calcium in the extracellular fluid inhibit the uptake of amino acids by chief cells, the synthesis of pre–pro-parathyroid hormone, its conversion to parathyroid hormone, and the release of the hormone into the circulation. Decreased levels of calcium have an opposite effect. The levels of phosphate range from 3 to 4.5 mg/dl (1.0 to 1.4 mmol/l) with approximately 15 percent bound to protein. However, the levels of phosphorus have no direct regulatory effects on the biosynthesis and secretion of parathyroid hormone.

Parathyroid hormone maintains serum calcium levels by directly or indirectly promoting calcium entry into the blood from bone, kidney, and the gastrointestinal tract (12,25). The hormone has a major action on bone which results ultimately in the inhibition of bone formation and the stimulation of bone resorption. Recent studies have shown that osteoblasts, but not osteoclasts, have receptors for parathyroid hormone. Although an increase in osteoclasts explains much of the bone resorbing activity of parathyroid hormone, the effects of the hormone on these cells is indirect and must be mediated by osteoblasts. Parathyroid hormone also has an important stimulatory effect on the cells that line endosteal surfaces. By stimulating renal synthesis of calcitriol, parathyroid hormone favors gastrointestinal absorption of calcium. In the kidney, parathyroid hormone stimulates tubular reabsorption of calcium, enhances clearance of phosphate, and promotes an increase in the enzyme that is important in the production of active vitamin D. These effects are mediated by the ability of parathyroid hormone to activate membrane-bound adenyl cyclases, leading to the generation of cyclic AMP.

Calcitriol is active in the same organs as parathyroid hormone (14,25). Calcitriol stimulates the absorption of calcium and phosphorus in the gut, inhibits the synthesis of pre–pro-parathyroid hormone, and enhances the mobilization of calcium stores from bone by increasing the numbers and activities of osteoclasts. In the kidney, calcitriol enhances renal reabsorption of phosphorus.

Calcitonin is a 32 amino acid peptide which is released from the thyroid when plasma calcium levels are increased. When administered to experimental animals with high bone turnover or to patients with Paget disease of bone, calcitonin results in a fall in plasma calcium levels. This effect is mediated by the inhibition of osteoclastic activity. The major physiologic role of calcitonin is most likely related to the protection of the skeleton during periods of calcium stress, including growth, pregnancy, and lactation (19).

ABNORMAL PHYSIOLOGY

HYPERCALCEMIA

Primary hyperparathyroidism and malignancy account for almost 90 percent of cases of hypercalcemia (19). Clinical features are helpful in the differential diagnosis of hypercalcemia. Generally, the finding of hypercalcemia in an asymptomatic adult usually suggests primary hyperparathyroidism, particularly if the hypercalcemia has been present for 1 or 2 years (9). Most patients with hypercalcemia associated with malignancy generally present with evidence of tumor although in a small number of instances the malignancy may remain occult.

HYPERPARATHYROIDISM

The term hyperparathyroidism refers to a metabolic derangement which is characterized by increased production of parathyroid hormone (2,9,10). Serum calcium may be low, normal, or high depending on a variety of other factors, such as renal function (15). In *primary hyperparathyroidism*, excess parathyroid hormone originates from an adenoma, hyperplasia, or carcinoma of the parathyroids and the serum calcium is typically increased, although occasional patients may have normocalcemic hyperparathyroidism. *Secondary hyperparathyroidism* refers to an adaptive increase of parathyroid hormone production induced most commonly by hypocalcemia and hyperphosphatemia associated with renal failure (14). *Tertiary hyperparathyroidism* refers to the development of apparent autonomous parathyroid hyperfunction in individuals with secondary hyperparathyroidism.

Primary Hyperparathyroidism

Primary hyperparathyroidism is a common disorder with an incidence that has increased dramatically over the past several decades. As a result, surgical exploration of the parathyroids has become a relatively commonplace procedure at most large institutions. Yet, the interpretation of the pathology of the parathyroids has generated considerable controversy and confusion with respect to the diagnostic criteria essential for the proper classification and treatment of patients with proliferative disorders of these endocrine glands.

Solitary adenomas are responsible for 80 to 85 percent of cases of hyperparathyroidism; this incidence has remained remarkably constant over the past 60 years (2). Parathyroid carcinomas, on the other hand, are rare neoplasms, accounting for not more than 2 to 3 percent of cases of primary hyperparathyroidism. Chief cell hyperplasia is responsible for the remaining cases. Clear cell hyperplasia is rare and appears to be decreasing in incidence although the reasons for this are not entirely clear.

The advent of multiphasic biochemical screening programs that include serum calcium and phosphorus determinations has had a major impact on the diagnosis of primary hyperparathyroidism and its mode of clinical presentation (22,23). The prevalence of primary hyperparathyroidism is considerably higher than was recognized earlier. Heath and co-workers (10) reported that the annual incidence per 100,000 population was only 7.8 between 1965 and 1974 but 51.1 between 1974 and 1976. In patients under the age of 40, the incidence is 10 cases per 100,000, while in males over 60 years of age the incidence is 92 per 100,000. In women older than 60, there are 188 cases per 100,000 population.

Many patients with mild hypercalcemia associated with hyperparathyroidism will not have any clinical manifestations of the disease, and only a relatively small proportion will develop a more severe form of hyperparathyroidism. However, there are no clinical or biochemical features that will predict such progression (27).

Prior to 1970, most patients with primary hyperparathyroidism presented with renal disease (calculi, nephrocalcinosis) or bone disorders (osteitis fibrosa cystica). More recently, however, almost half of the patients have been asymptomatic or have relatively mild and nonspecific complaints of weakness and lethargy (10).

Approaches to the treatment of hyperparathyroidism are becoming generally well established. Most large case series indicate that patients do well with excision only of abnormal glands and that routine subtotal parathyroidectomy does not substantially improve cure rates.

Bone Changes. While osteitis fibrosa cystica is decreasing in incidence, the frequency of simple diffuse osteopenia resembling osteoporosis is increasing in patients with hyperparathyroidism (2,10,24). This phenomenon may be related to the earlier detection of hyperparathyroidism. Patients with hyperparathyroidism have a statistically higher incidence of diffuse osteopenia of the spine, with associated crush fractures, as compared to age- and sex-matched controls. Metabolic studies have revealed increased rates of bone turnover in affected patients. In addition to osteopenia, patients with hyperparathyroidism may manifest a variety of articular and periarticular disorders. These include chondrocalcinosis with or without attacks of pseudogout, juxta-articular erosions, subchondral fractures, traumatic synovitis, calcific periarthritis, and true gout.

Bone changes in patients with hyperparathyroidism range from mild diffuse osteopenia to large lytic lesions characterized by fibrosis, hemosiderin deposition, and giant cell formation (fig. 13) (2). Lytic lesions, which have a propensity to develop within the jaws, calvarium, and long tubular bones, have been referred to as "brown tumors" or *osteitis fibrosa cystica generalisata* (von Recklinghausen disease).

The earliest phases of bone disease in patients with hyperparathyroidism are characterized by osteoclastic resorption of subperiosteal and endosteal bone surfaces and replacement of resorbed bone by fibrous tissue. A characteristic feature is the presence of dissecting osteitis; the bone trabeculae are hollowed out by osteoclasts and are replaced by fibrous tissue (fig. 14). The finding of

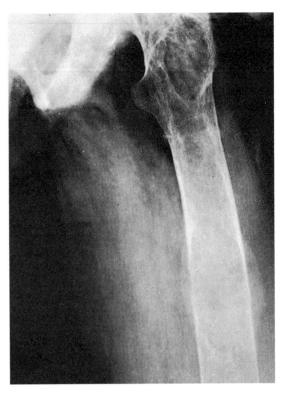

Figure 13
OSTEITIS FIBROSA CYSTICA GENERALISATA
This X ray of a femur shows generalized osteopenia and multiple cysts. (Fig. 7 from Fascicle 15, First Series.)

dissecting osteitis is virtually diagnostic of hyperparathyroidism.

The development of brown tumors begins with resorption of bone trabecula (figs. 14–17). The fibrous response may develop as a consequence of microfractures within partially resorbed bone, followed by bleeding, hemosiderin deposition, and the accumulation of giant cells. With further hemorrhage, cystic degeneration ultimately occurs. Giant cells, including osteoclasts and foreign body giant cells, are often aggregated in nodular foci around areas of hemosiderin deposition. Areas of osteoid formation and reactive woven bone may be prominent in some brown tumors.

Both brown tumors and giant cell reparative granulomas frequently involve the jaws, and the histologic differentiation of these entities is impossible. The giant cells found in true giant cell tumors tend to be more evenly spaced than those in brown tumors (fig. 18), the stromal cells tend to be plumper, and osteoblastic activity is less conspicuous.

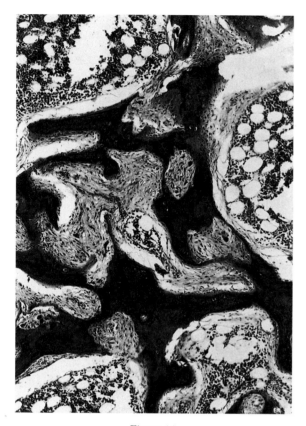

Figure 14
DISSECTING OSTEITIS
In this bone biopsy showing dissecting osteitis the trabecula are invaded by fibrous tissue.

Ultrastructural studies of brown tumors have revealed that the giant cells have features similar to inactive osteoclasts, including numerous mitochondria, dilated endoplasmic reticulum, perinuclear Golgi regions, sparse lysosomes, and short filopodia (5). In contrast to active osteoclasts, the giant cells lack prominent ruffled borders. The stromal compartment includes cells with the ultrastructural features of fibroblasts, myofibroblasts, and histiocytes.

In secondary hyperparathyroidism, there is evidence of osteomalacia with widened osteoid seams, together with superimposed osteoclastic activity, including the presence of dissecting osteitis.

Other Changes. Recurrent nephrolithiasis has been reported in 5 to 20 percent of patients with primary hyperparathyroidism in a recent series as compared to 70 percent in an earlier series (10). In addition to the presence of calculi, renal disease may be manifested by increased blood urea nitrogen and creatinine, decreased glomerular filtration rate, and a wide variety of renal tubular defects including reduced net acid secretion, aminoaciduria, and glycosuria.

Neuromuscular manifestations include fatigability and weakness, primarily with involvement of the proximal musculature (10). Surgical treatment of the hyperparathyroidism has resulted in amelioration of these symptoms in a significant

Figure 15
OSTEITIS FIBROSA
CYSTICA
GENERALISATA

The right portion of the field shows loose fibrous connective tissue with reactive new bone formation. The central area shows hemorrhage in fibrous tissue and cyst formation. (Fig. 5 from Fascicle 15, First Series.)

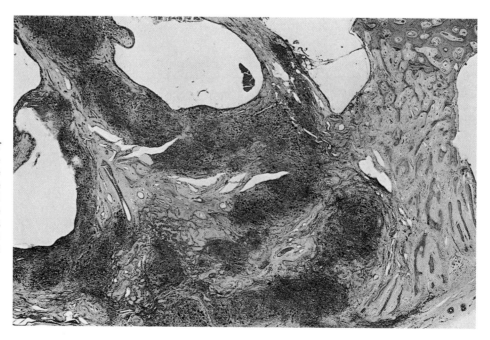

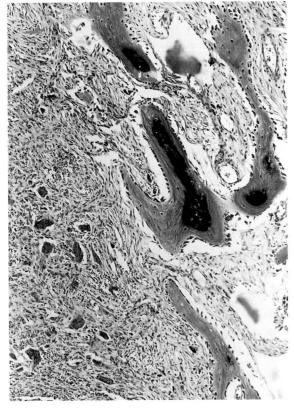

Figure 16
BROWN TUMOR
Peripheral region of brown tumor with reactive bone formation. The brown tumor consists of stromal elements and dispersed giant cells.

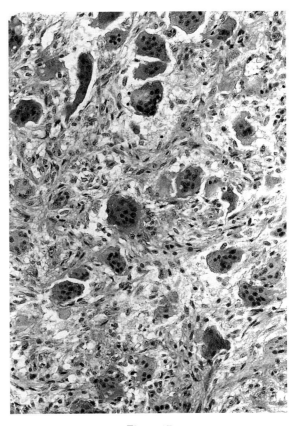

Figure 17
BROWN TUMOR
This central region of brown tumor shows giant cells separated by plump stromal cells.

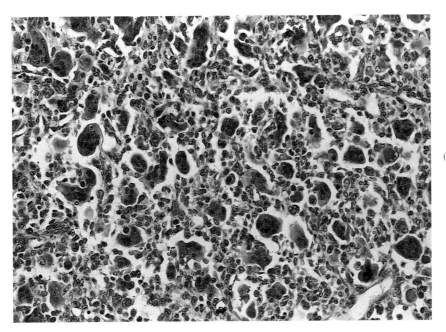

Figure 18
GIANT CELL BONE TUMOR
True giant cell tumor of bone (compare with fig. 15).

proportion of affected patients. Psychiatric symptoms include personality changes, depression, and psychomotor retardation. Rarely, coma has occurred in patients with hyperparathyroidism.

Gastrointestinal disorders include peptic ulcer, abdominal distress, pancreatic calcifications, acute and chronic pancreatitis, constipation, and vomiting. Ocular signs include band keratopathy, conjunctivitis, and deposits of calcium within the conjunctiva. Hypertension has also been reported in patients with hyperthyroidism.

Laboratory Diagnosis. Primary hyperparathyroidism may be defined as the excessive secretion of parathyroid hormone in the absence of an appropriate physiological stimulus (8,15,25). Uncomplicated primary hyperparathyroidism is typically associated with elevated serum calcium and decreased serum inorganic phosphorus. The decreased concentration of inorganic phosphorus results primarily from parathyroid hormone–induced phosphate diuresis caused by decreased renal tubular reabsorption.

Since the regulated component of serum calcium is that portion not bound to plasma protein, serum calcium levels should be normalized to plasma protein concentrations (19). Measurements of ionized serum calcium levels present the greatest diagnostic sensitivity. Detection of excess phosphate diuresis is sometimes helpful in distinguishing hyperparathyroidism from other causes of hypercalcemia. This can be achieved by measuring tubular reabsorption of phosphate or renal phosphate clearance. In hyperparathyroidism, tubular reabsorption of phosphate is less than 78 percent, while phosphate clearance is greater than 18 ml/min. Patients with primary hyperparathyroidism and humoral hypercalcemia of malignancy also generally have increased urinary cyclic AMP levels.

Measurements of serum levels of parathyroid hormone by radioimmunoassay have been difficult because of the heterogeneity of the circulating hormone (20,28). Subsequent to its secretion from the parathyroid gland, parathyroid hormone is cleaved at position 34, primarily in the liver, to yield an amino terminal molecule with a short half-life but potent biological activity and a carboxy terminal fragment with a longer half-life but little or no biological activity. In patients with normal renal function, intact parathyroid hormone comprises most of the parathyroid hormone–like bio-

Table 1

SECONDARY HYPERPARATHYROIDISM

Chronic renal failure

Dietary deficiency of vitamin D or calcium

Malabsorption syndromes

Tissue resistance to vitamin D

Severe hypomagnesemia

Pseudohypoparathyroidism

activity; the N-terminal fragment comprises up to 60 percent of the bioactivity in individuals with chronic renal failure. Clearance of the various parathyroid hormone fragments is impaired in individuals with chronic renal failure.

Most radioimmunoassays for parathyroid hormone utilize antisera which recognize N-terminal, C-terminal, or midportions of the molecule (28); newer assays recognize intact parathyroid hormone. In these assays, N-terminal antiserum is used to extract peptides bearing the amino terminus, followed by a second antiserum which recognizes the midportion of the molecule. These assays, therefore, measure only N-terminal fragments attached to an intact sequence of the midportion of the molecule. The reference value for the intact parathyroid hormone molecule is 210–310 pg/ml.

Secondary and Tertiary Hyperparathyroidism

Secondary hyperparathyroidism (Table 1) is characterized by an increased production of parathyroid hormone, most commonly as a result of hypocalcemia and hyperphosphatemia (8,9,26). Hypocalcemia leads to stimulation of parathyroid function and hyperplasia of the glands .

Secondary hyperparathyroidism occurs in patients with renal failure, vitamin D deficiency, and pseudohypoparathyroidism which is characterized by a subnormal response to parathyroid hormone at the level of the receptor. There is an adaptive increase in gland size in secondary hyperparathyroidism while the growth of the parathyroid in primary hyperparathyroidism is autonomous.

The term tertiary hyperparathyroidism refers to the development of apparent autonomous hyperparathyroidism in patients with proven pre-existing secondary hyperparathyroidism (26).

Familial Hyperparathyroidism

Familial hyperparathyroidism occurs most commonly in association with multiple endocrine neoplastic syndromes (10), but can also occur in the absence of other endocrine abnormalities. Affected patients generally have evidence of parathyroid chief cell hyperplasia.

Neonatal Hyperparathyroidism

Hyperparathyroidism in the neonate is rare. Affected infants appear normal at birth; symptoms associated with severe hypercalcemia generally become evident within the first week of life. Skeletal X rays show severe demineralization, subperiosteal resorption, and pathologic fractures (1). Renal calcinosis may also be evident on plain films of the abdomen.

Recent studies suggest that this type of hyperparathyroidism is related to familial benign (hypocalciuric) hypercalcemia. It has also been suggested that neonates affected with this syndrome may have two copies of the abnormal gene. Neonatal hyperparathyroidism is considered a surgical emergency, since most affected infants die between 2 and 7 months if untreated (1). Total parathyroidectomy is the treatment of choice because of the high rate of recurrence following subtotal parathyroidectomy. The resected glands usually show evidence of diffuse hyperplasia.

Neonatal hyperparathyroidism may also occur in infants born to mothers with surgical hypoparathyroidism or poorly treated idiopathic hypoparathyroidism (1).

OTHER CAUSES OF HYPERCALCEMIA

Malignancy-Associated Hypercalcemia

Malignancy related causes of hypercalcemia are shown in Table 2 (12,18). In patients with extensive bone metastases or myeloma associated with extensive skeletal destruction, hypercalcemia most likely results from the local release of bone resorbing substances directly from the tumor (localized osteolytic hypercalcemia).

Table 2

TUMORS ASSOCIATED WITH HYPERCALCEMIA

A. Humoral Hypercalcemia of Malignancy	
Site	**Tumor Type**
Lung	Squamous cell carcinoma
Esophagus	Squamous cell carcinoma
Head and neck	Squamous cell carcinoma
Vulva, vagina, cervix	Squamous cell carcinoma
Kidney	Renal (clear) cell carcinoma, transitional cell carcinoma of pelvis
Urinary bladder	Transitional cell carcinoma
Ovary	Small cell carcinoma, clear cell carcinoma
Liver	Hepatocellular carcinoma, cholangiocarcinoma
Pancreas	Islet cell neoplasms, ductal adenocarcinoma
Colon	Adenocarcinoma

B. Localized Osteolytic Hypercalcemia	
Site	**Tumor Type**
Breast	Adenocarcinoma
Lymphoreticular	Malignant lymphoma
Bone	Multiple myeloma

Numerous factors including transforming growth factors (TGFs), interleukins, and tumor necrosis factor, have been implicated in the development of localized osteolytic hypercalcemia (12,18,30). TGF alpha, which belongs to the epidermal growth factor family, stimulates osteoclastic resorption of bone in organ culture and inhibits the function of osteoblasts. The role of TGF beta in the genesis of localized osteolytic hypercalcemia is less clear, and its action appears to be mediated by prostaglandins.

Interleukin-1, which is produced by activated monocytes, has multiple biological actions, including osteoclastic bone resorption. This substance has also been referred to as osteoclast-activating factor. Interleukin-1 alpha acts synergistically with factors that act via the parathyroid hormone receptor and with TGF alpha. Tumor necrosis factor, as well as a variety of colony-stimulating factors, may also be involved with tumor-mediated bone resorption. In some instances, prostaglandins may have a role in local bone resorption by tumors.

Hypercalcemia occurring in the absence of extensive skeletal metastases has been referred to as *pseudohyperparathyroidism* or as the *syndrome of humoral hypercalcemia of malignancy*. Although early studies had suggested that this syndrome was mediated by the ectopic secretion of parathyroid hormone, recent studies indicate that the likely candidate for this syndrome is parathyroid hormone–related protein (PTHRP) (12). The gene encoding PTHRP is a complex transcriptional unit which, by alternate splicing, gives rise to messenger RNAs that encode three related PTHRPs. The PTHRP gene has been localized to chromosome 12 (1a).

PTHRP has a molecular weight of 16,000 to 17,000 daltons. The amino terminal portion of the molecule shows considerable sequence homology with parathyroid hormone. In addition to its presence in a variety of tumors, PTHRP has been found in normal keratinocytes, parathyroid glands, lactating mammary glands, placenta, and other sites. PTHRP interacts with parathyroid hormone receptors and can cause hypercalcemia when infused into experimental animals. In patients with the syndrome of humoral hypercalcemia of malignancy, there is evidence of intense bone resorption and increased renal tubular calcium absorption. In contrast to patients with localized osteolytic hypercalcemia, nephrogenic cyclic AMP levels are typically increased. In addition, immunoreactive parathyroid hormone and 1,25 dihydroxyvitamin D are suppressed (1a).

The tumors most commonly associated with the syndrome of humoral hypercalcemia of malignancy include renal cell carcinomas and squamous cell carcinomas of the upper and lower respiratory tracts (Table 2) (21,29). In addition, transitional and squamous cell carcinomas of the renal pelvis and urinary bladder, and squamous cell carcinomas of the vulva, vagina, and cervix have been implicated.

Approximately 50 percent of the cases of hypercalcemia associated with ovarian tumors have been identified in patients with small cell carcinomas, while clear cell carcinomas have accounted for the remaining cases (6). Humoral hypercalcemia of malignancy has also been noted in patients with hepatocellular carcinoma, cholangiocarcinoma, and pheochromocytoma (29). In the pediatric population, the syndrome has been seen in association with Wilms tumor and rhabdomyosarcoma.

Familial Benign (Hypocalciuric) Hypercalcemia

Familial benign (hypocalciuric) hypercalcemia is an uncommon but important hereditary disorder characterized by hypercalcemia occurring early in life and an autosomal dominant pattern of inheritance (11,16). Affected patients typically have mild hypercalcemia, hypermagnesemia, variable hypophosphatemia, normal serum parathyroid hormone levels, and low urinary excretion of calcium relative to serum calcium. Serum calcium values in affected individuals tend to be highest in infancy and decline in childhood and adulthood.

Thorgeirsson and co-workers (31) reported that the parathyroid glands of patients with familial benign hypercalcemia are enlarged and show evidence of increased parathyroid parenchymal area. Other authors, however, have not confirmed these observations. In the series of cases reported by Law and co-workers (13), 80 percent of the glands were within normal limits for weight and the parenchymal area was less than that of age-matched controls. The remaining cases in Law's series had increased parathyroid weight but most were indistinguishable from normal glands. The finding of minimally enlarged parathyroid glands in patients with hypercalcemia should suggest the possibility of familial benign hypercalcemia. Subtotal parathyroidectomy is not advisable.

Although there are no consistent histologic abnormalities in familial benign hypercalcemia, it is clear that the glands are functionally abnormal. Analyses of parathyroid function in these patients suggest that there may be a reset error in which calcium sensitivity of chief cells is retained at a supranormal level. It is also possible that the kidneys in affected patients are hypersensitive to the effects of parathyroid hormone.

Although familial benign (hypocalciuric) hypercalcemia is inherited as an autosomal dominant trait, individuals with two copies of the gene have life-threatening hypercalcemia and severe parathyroid hyperplasia, evident at birth (16,17).

Lithium-Associated Hypercalcemia

Approximately 10 percent of patients on lithium will have hypercalcemia mediated by the parathyroid glands and accompanied by increased levels of parathyroid hormone (9,14,19). Rarely, some patients with lithium-associated hypercalcemia may have parathyroid adenomas but this association is probably coincidental. In most instances, the hypercalcemia disappears following cessation of lithium treatment.

Other Hypercalcemic Syndromes

Vitamin D related causes of hypercalcemia include vitamin D intoxication, sarcoidosis and other granulomatous disorders, and the idiopathic hypercalcemia of infancy which is due to abnormal vitamin D sensitivity (19). Disorders associated with high bone turnover and hypercalcemia include hyperthyroidism, immobilization, thiazide diuretics, and vitamin A intoxication.

PARATHYROID GLANDS IN NONPARATHYROID HORMONE-MEDIATED HYPERCALCEMIA

Occasional patients with nonparathyroid related causes of hypercalcemia will undergo surgical exploration of the parathyroids for suspected hyperparathyroidism. In most cases, the parathyroids are normal in size and show some decrease in the amount of stromal fat. Since some of these cases include patients with malignancy-associated hypercalcemia, it is likely that the decreased stromal fat results from poor nutritional status.

Dufour and colleagues (7) studied the parathyroids of 12 patients with hypercalcemia of diverse etiologies. The glands in these patients were similar to normals in size and fat to parenchyma ratio. All glands had a normal parenchymal cross-sectional area calculated as the product of gland area and parenchymal fraction.

Histologic study revealed that the glands were composed of small dark chief cells arranged in cords and nests. Occasional chief cells had more abundant pale-staining cytoplasm with numerous vacuoles and a peripherally displaced nucleus. The vacuolated cells tended to be arranged in a trabecular pattern, particularly at the periphery of the gland. Examination of the glands with Sudan IV stains revealed focal intracellular fat. These findings indicate that the parathyroid glands of patients with nonparathyroid hormone-mediated hypercalcemia are similar to normal glands in most respects.

REFERENCES

1. Anast CS. Disorders of mineral and bone metabolism. In: Avery ME, Taeusch TW, eds. Schaffer's diseases of the newborn. 5th ed. Philadelphia: WB Saunders, 1984:464–79.

1a. Capen CC, Rosol TJ. Pathobiology of parathyroid hormone and parathyroid hormone-related protein. In: LiVolsi VA, DeLellis RA, eds. Pathobiology of the parathyroid and thyroid glands. Baltimore: Williams and Wilkins, 1993:1–33.

2. Castleman B, Roth SI. Tumors of the parathyroid glands. Atlas of Tumor Pathology, 2nd Series, Fascicle 14. Washington, D.C.: Armed Forces Institute of Pathology, 1978;1–94.

3. Cohn DV, MacGregor RR. The biosynthesis, intracellular processing and secretion of parahormone. Endocr Rev 1981;2:1–26.

4. _____, Morrissey JJ, Shofstall RE, Chu LL. Cosecretion of secretory protein-I and parathormone by dispersed bovine parathyroid cells. Endocrinology 1982; 110:625–30.

5. Desai P, Steiner GC. Ultrastructure of brown tumor of hyperparathyroidism. Ultrastruct Pathol 1990;14:505–11.

6. Dickersin GR, Kline IW, Scully RE. Small cell carcinoma of the ovary with hypercalcemia. A report of 11 cases. Cancer 1982;49:188–97.

7. Dufour DR, Marx SJ, Spiegel AM. Parathyroid gland morphology in non-parathyroid hormone-mediated hypercalcemia. Am J Surg Pathol 1985;9:43–51.

8. Endres DB, Villanueva R, Sharp CF Jr, Singer FR. Measurement of parathyroid hormone. Endocrinol Metab Clin North Am 1989;18:611–29.

9. Greenspan FS. Basic and clinical endocrinology. Norwalk, Conn: Appleton and Lange, 1991.

10. Heath DA. Primary hyperparathyroidism. Clinical presentation and factors influencing clinical management. Endocrinol Metab Clin North Am 1989;18:631–46.

11. Heath H III. Familial benign (hypocalciuric) hypercalcemia. A troublesome mimic of mild primary hyperparathyroidism. Endocrinol Metab Clin North Am 1989;18:723–40.

12. Insogna KL. Humoral hypercalcemia of malignancy. The role of parathyroid hormone-related protein. Endocrinol Metab Clin North Am 1989;18:779–94.

13. Law WM Jr., Carney JA, Heath H III. Parathyroid glands in familial benign hypercalcemia (familial hypocalciuric hypercalcemia). Am J Med 1984;76:1021–6.

14. Mallette LE. Regulation of blood calcium in humans. Endocrinol Metab Clin North Am 1989;18:601–10.

15. Marcus R. Laboratory diagnosis of primary hyperparathyroidism. Endocrinol Metab Clin North Am 1989;18: 647–58.

16. Marx SJ. Genetic defects in primary hyperparathyroidism [Editorial]. N Engl J Med 1988;318:699–701.

17. Matsuo M, Okita K, Takemine H, Fujita T. Neonatal primary hyperparathyroidism in familial hypocalciuric hypercalcemia. Am J Dis Child 1982;136:728–31.

18. Mundy GR. Hypercalcemic factors other than parathyroid hormone related protein. Endocrinol Metab Clin North Am 1989;18:795–806.

19. Neer RM. Calcium and inorganic phosphate homeostasis. In: DeGroot LJ, ed. Endocrinology, Vol. 2. 2nd ed. Philadelphia: WB Saunders, 1989:927–53.

20. Nussbaum SR, Zahradnik RJ, Lavigne JR, et al. Highly sensitive two-site immunoradiometric assay of parathyrin and its clinical utility in evaluating patients with hypercalcemia. Clin Chem 1987;33:1364–7.

21. Omenn GS, Roth SI, Baker WH. Hyperparathyroidism associated with malignant tumors of nonparathyroid origin. Cancer 1969;24:1004–11.

22. Palmér M, Jakobsson S, Akerström G, Ljunghall S. Prevalence of hypercalcemia in a health survey: a 14-year follow-up study of serum calcium values. Eur J Clin Invest 1988;18:39–46.

23. _____, Ljunghall S, Akerström G, et al. Patients with primary hyperparathyroidism operated on over a 24-year period: temporal trends of clinical and laboratory findings. J Chronic Dis 1987;40:121–30.

24. Parisien M, Silverberg SJ, Shane E, Dempster DW, Bilezikian JP. Bone disease in primary hyperparathyroidism. Endocrinol Metab Clin North Am 1990;19:19–34.

25. Rosenblatt M, Kronenberg HM, Potts JT Jr. Parathyroid hormone. Physiology, chemistry, biosynthesis, secretion, metabolism and mode of action. In: DeGroot LJ, ed. Endocrinology, Vol. 2. 2nd ed. Philadelphia: WB Saunders, 1989:848–91.

26. Salusky IB, Coburn JW. The renal osteodystrophies. In: DeGroot LJ, ed. Endocrinology, Vol. 2. 2nd ed. Philadelphia: WB Saunders, 1989:1032–48.

27. Scholz DA, Purnell DC. Asymptomatic primary hyperparathyroidism: ten year prospective study. Mayo Clin Proc 1981;56:473–8.

28. Segre GV, Potts JT Jr. Differential diagnosis of hypercalcemia: methods and clinical applications of parathyroid assays. In: DeGroot LJ, ed. Endocrinology, Vol. 2. 2nd ed. Philadelphia: WB Saunders, 1989:948–1001.

29. Skrabanek P, McPartlin J, Powell D. Tumor hypercalcemia and "ectopic hyperparathyroidism." Medicine (Baltimore) 1980,59:262–82.

30. Stewart AF, Insogna K, Broadus AE. Malignancy associated hypercalcemia. In: DeGroot LJ, ed. Endocrinology, Vol. 2. 2nd ed. Philadelphia: WB Saunders, 1989:967–83.

31. Thorgeirsson U, Costa J, Marx SJ. The parathyroid glands in familial hypocalciuric hypercalcemia. Hum Pathol 1981;12:229–37.

✧✧✧

PARATHYROID ADENOMA

Definition. A benign neoplasm composed of chief cells, oncocytic cells, transitional oncocytic cells, or mixtures of these cell types. In the vast majority of cases, adenomas involve a single parathyroid gland.

General Features. Parathyroid adenoma is the single most common cause of primary hyperparathyroidism. However, there is considerable variation in the incidence of adenomas as reported from different institutions, ranging from 25 to 96 percent (17,29). This variation undoubtedly reflects both lack of uniformity of diagnostic criteria and differences in patterns of patient referral. For example, those institutions having a large proportion of patients with one of the familial hyperparathyroidism syndromes will have a higher incidence of patients with diagnoses of hyperplasia.

In most large case series, approximately 80 percent of all patients with primary hyperparathyroidism have a single parathyroid adenoma (17). While adenomas can occur at any age, most become evident in the fourth decade. Parathyroid adenomas occur more commonly in females with a ratio of about 3 to 1.

The precise histopathologic definition of parathyroid adenoma, however, has remained elusive. In their seminal study of the pathology of hyperparathyroidism, Castleman and Mallory (16) stressed the localized character of the proliferative process in cases of adenoma, noting that it was limited not only to a single gland but often to a portion of a single gland. Further support for the concept of the neoplastic origin of the adenoma was based on the demonstration of an adjacent rim of normal parathyroid tissue in 8 of their 19 cases. The lack of recurrent hyperparathyroidism after removal of the single enlarged gland was additional evidence for the neoplastic origin of their cases.

Some studies, however, have suggested that parathyroid adenomas represent localized hyperplasias of chief cells. In a study of 172 cases of primary hyperparathyroidism, Ghandur-Mnaymneh and Kimura (29) concluded that hyperplasia with single gland involvement was responsible for 75 percent of cases. This conclu-

sion was based on the use of three histologic criteria for the diagnosis of hyperplasia: 1) presence of fat cells within the proliferation; 2) lack of sharp delineation between the proliferation and adjacent parathyroid tissue; and 3) retention of the lobular pattern of the normal parathyroid. The rarity of recurrent hyperparathyroidism following removal of a single gland was explained by the slow progression of the disease and the focal nature of the hyperplastic process.

If adenomas did, in fact, represent hyperplasias rather than neoplastic proliferations, one would expect the cells to be polyclonal. Early studies that employed isoenzymes of glucose-6-phosphate dehydrogenase suggested that most parathyroid adenomas were polyclonal proliferations (34). However, more recent studies employing molecular approaches have established that parathyroid adenomas, and some hyperplasias, represent clonal proliferations (8,25,44). These studies are based on the demonstration of clonal rearrangements of the parathyroid hormone gene, analysis of the X-linked hypoxanthine phosphoribosyl-transferase gene, or the presence of consistent chromosomal abnormalities. These studies suggest that the underlying abnormality in DNA structure originated in one cell as a rare event, such as a somatic mutation. Friedman and co-workers (25) found losses of alleles from chromosome 11 in 26 percent of sporadic parathyroid adenomas and in most of these cases, the losses involved the region of the putative multiple endocrine neoplasia (MEN) I gene.

Several reports (4,31,36), however, suggest that some adenomas may arise from preexisting hyperplasias. Akerström and co-workers (4) performed a detailed analysis of parathyroid glands obtained at autopsy from 422 patients. None of the patients had clinical, biochemical, or histologic evidence of advanced renal disease. Parathyroid hyperplasia, based on total parenchymal weights in excess of 144 mg, was identified in 7 percent of cases while adenomas were found in 2.4 percent. The hyperplastic glands were frequently nodular and asymmetric with increased numbers of oncocytic cells and chief cells. Some of the largest hyperplastic nodules were indistinguishable from adenomas.

Analysis of serum calcium levels revealed elevations in subjects with adenomas and hyperplastic glands containing large nodules. On the basis of these observations, Akerström and co-workers concluded that nodularity of parathyroid tissue is a sign of abnormality and that adenomas may arise from foci of nodular hyperplasia. This concept is supported in part by a molecular study (25) that demonstrated clonal loss of alleles from chromosome 11 in 10 of 16 enlarged (histologically hyperplastic) parathyroid glands in patients with MEN I. Lesions with chromosome losses were generally larger than those without, and these findings have suggested that a monoclonal "adenoma" may develop from a phase of polyclonal hyperplasia.

The existence of double or multiple adenomas as a cause of primary hyperparathyroidism has been a subject of controversy (33). Verdonk and Edis (66) reported double adenomas in 38 of 1,962 patients (1.9 percent) with primary hyperparathyroidism. The criteria for inclusion in this study included: (1) excision of two enlarged and hypercellular glands each weighing more than 70 mg and (2) the identification and preservation of two other normal sized parathyroids. In this group, the mean age was 54 years. Five of the patients had one of the MEN syndromes, but there were no patients with isolated familial hyperparathyroidism. Following surgical treatment, 37 patients had normal parathyroid function with an average follow-up of 4.6 years. Only one of the 5 patients with MEN had persistent hypercalcemia; the others were cured of their hypercalcemia. While some of these cases may be multiple adenomas, most are probably asymmetric or pseudoadenomatous hyperplasia.

There are few data relating to the pathogenesis of parathyroid adenomas. These tumors may occur in association with types I and II MEN syndromes (5,17,27,40). More often, however, the parathyroid lesions in the MEN syndromes are classified histologically as chief cell hyperplasia rather than adenoma.

There is some evidence to support the role of ionizing irradiation in the development of parathyroid adenomas. Several studies have indicated that primary hyperparathyroidism and thyroid cancer occur together more often than expected by chance alone (42,47). In a series of 12 patients with coexistent well-differentiated thyroid carcinoma and primary hyperparathyroidism, 8 were found to have had prior radiation exposure to the head and neck, including 1 patient who received ^{131}I for thyroid cancer; Tisell and co-workers (65) found that 15 percent of 170 patients with hyperparathyroidism had received prior irradiation to the head and neck; Prinz and co-workers (53) showed that 30 percent of patients studied had received prior irradiation; and in a series of 74 consecutive patients with parathyroid adenomas, Russ and co-workers (60) reported that 25 percent gave a history of prior radiation exposure.

Clinical Features. The laboratory findings in patients with parathyroid adenoma do not differ from patients with other types of primary hyperparathyroidism. Parathyroid adenomas are rarely large enough to produce a palpable mass (17,48).

There are numerous approaches to the preoperative localization of parathyroid adenomas including CT scanning, venography with selective sampling for parathyroid hormone levels, selenomethionine or thallium 201 scanning, and thermography (48). The success rates of CT scanning, radioactive thallium scanning, and ultrasonography have ranged from 60 to 90 percent in previously unoperated cases. In patients with recurrent hyperparathyroidism following an initial surgical procedure, selective venous catheterization with parathyroid hormone radioimmunoassays provides the highest yield for localization of abnormal parathyroid tissue.

Gross Findings. Parathyroid adenomas may occur at any site in which normal parathyroid tissue is found (16,17,22,70) (pl. III–VI). Approximately 90 percent of all adenomas involve the upper or lower glands of the neck, with the lower glands more frequently involved. The remaining 10 percent occur in a variety of other sites including the mediastinum (pl. VI), retroesophageal soft tissue, and within the thyroid or esophagus. Rarely, adenomas may arise from ectopic or supernumerary parathyroid tissue present within the pericardium, the vagus nerve, or soft tissue adjacent to the angle of the jaw (56). The incidence of parathyroid adenomas in these uncommon sites is relatively high in centers to which patients are referred for reoperations for persistent or recurrent hyperparathyroidism. For example, Cohn and Silen (19) found a 12 percent

PLATE III
PARATHYROID ADENOMAS

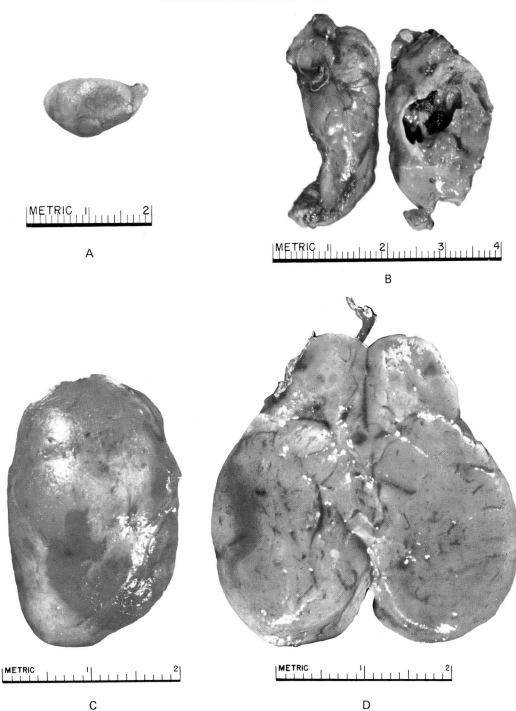

(Plates A and B from Fascicle 15, First Series; plates C and D from Fascicle 14, Second Series)

A.   Small orange-brown adenoma.
B.   External (left) and cross-sectional views (right) of 3 g cystic adenoma.
C.   Large orange-brown adenoma (4.2 g).
D.   Cross section of 2.7 g adenoma.

PLATE IV
PARATHYROID ADENOMA

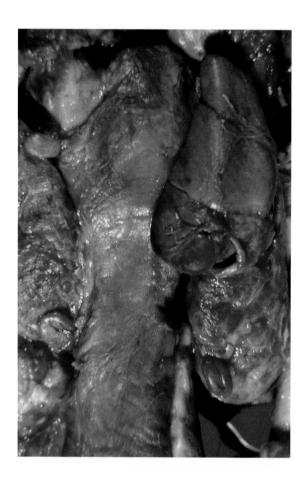

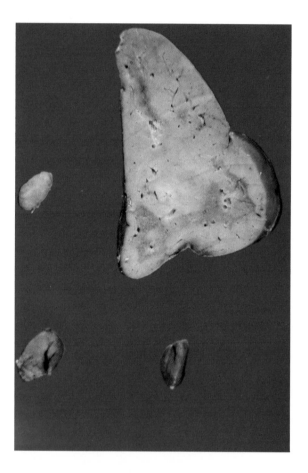

A. In situ postmortem dissection of parathyroid glands in a patient with primary hyperparathyroidism. The lobes of the thyroid have been reflected anteriorly. The right upper parathyroid is replaced by a large adenoma, which has a pyramidal shape and surface lobulations. The remaining three glands are normal. (Courtesy of Dr. Manfred Stolte, Bayreuth, Germany.)

B. Cross section of parathyroid adenoma shown in A. The remaining three glands are normal. (Courtesy of Dr. Manfred Stolte, Bayreuth, Germany.)

PLATE V

PARATHYROID ADENOMA

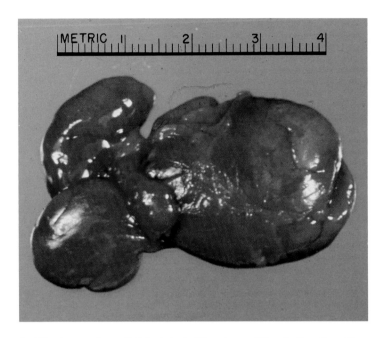

A. The tumor is multilobulated. (Courtesy of Dr. Arthur Lee, Burlington, MA.)

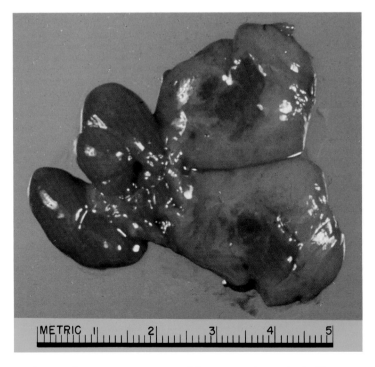

B. Orange-brown cross section of the tumor shown in A. (Courtesy of Dr. Arthur Lee, Burlington, MA.)

PLATE VI

MEDIASTINAL PARATHYROID ADENOMA

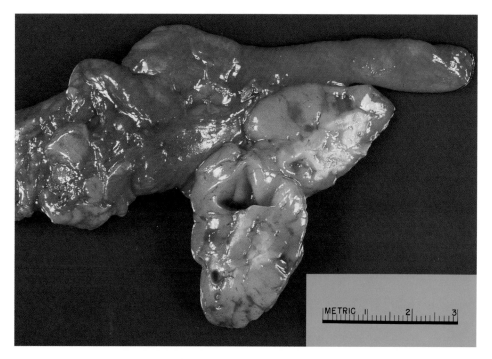

A. Left, thymus; right, bisected adenoma. The adenoma shows scattered cystic foci. (Courtesy of Dr. Byunku Chun, Washington, DC.)

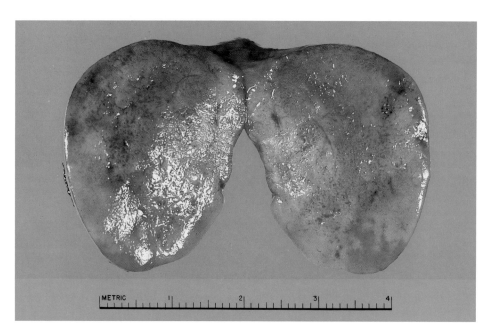

B. The tumor is well encapsulated and shows a homogeneous appearance on cut surface. (Courtesy of Dr. Byunku Chun, Washington, DC.)

incidence of intrathyroidal parathyroid adenomas in patients referred for reoperation.

The typical parathyroid adenoma is an encapsulated neoplasm which characteristically involves a single gland. The capsule is generally thin and this feature permits relatively easy surgical dissection of the adenoma from the adjacent thyroid and surrounding soft tissues in the neck.

Adenomas vary considerably in size. Microadenomas measure less than 6 mm in diameter (54). These lesions can be so small that they may be missed on surgical exploration and frozen section examinations (39). In several reported cases, microadenomas were apparent only after serially sectioning the paraffin-embedded blocks (39,54).

There is some correlation between the weight of the adenoma and the serum levels of calcium, parathyroid hormone concentration, and clinical symptomatology (3,17). In cases reported by the Massachusetts General Hospital (17), adenomas associated with severe bone disease had an average weight of 10 g, while the average adenoma weight in individuals without bone disease was 1.3 g, with many weighing less than 0.5 g.

Adenomas also vary considerably in shape. Large tumors are ovoid in configuration and are sharply separated from the surrounding adipose tissue. Occasionally, however, adenomas are elongated and have a bilobed or multilobed configuration (pls. IV, V) (16,17). The risk of incomplete excision is higher in adenomas with a multilobular configuration than in those with smooth contours.

Adenomas vary from tan to orange-brown (pl. III), and the consistency is usually soft. If an enlarged gland is suspected of being an adenoma, it is essential to confirm that the remaining glands are normal in size.

In the past, considerable stress was placed on the demonstration of an uninvolved rim of parathyroid tissue adjacent to the adenoma. However, such a rim is found in only 50 to 60 percent of proven adenoma cases. The rim of the normal gland, commonly found in the hilar region, is generally light brown or yellow, in contrast to the red-brown color of the adenoma. The absence of a rim of residual parathyroid tissue, however, does not exclude the diagnosis of adenoma.

In most cases, the cut surface of the adenoma appears homogeneous but nodularity may be evident (pl. V). Foci of cystic change are apparent in many cases, with individual cysts ranging from 0.1 to 1.0 cm in diameter. The cysts may be filled with clear to brown fluid. Cystic degeneration may be extreme and there may be foci of fibrosis, calcification, and hemosiderin deposition (16,17). Rarely, the walls of cystically degenerated adenomas are thickened and adherent to the surrounding soft tissues of the neck or thyroid. Occasionally, degeneration of an adenoma leads to complete cystification.

Microscopic Findings. The intraoperative diagnosis of parathyroid lesions together with a discussion of fat stains, fine-needle aspiration biopsy, flow cytometry, and density gradients is presented in Procedures for Pathologic Examination.

The vast majority of parathyroid adenomas are composed of closely packed chief cells at various stages of their secretory cycles (6,11,17,18). The cells are commonly arranged in cords and nests, glandular formations, or sheets with frequent admixtures of these patterns (figs. 19–29).

The dominant cell type within most adenomas is the chief cell (12,17). These cells are often larger than the chief cells present in the adjacent normal parathyroid tissue (figs. 19, 20, 22). Most cells within the adenoma are 8 to 14 μm in diameter and have a polyhedral shape with indistinct outlines. The cytoplasm is faintly eosinophilic but occasionally appears clear. In some instances, the cytoplasm appears vacuolated and some cells may have perinuclear halos (figs. 25, 27). Nodular aggregates of cells with more or less cytoplasm than the bulk of chief cells comprising the adenoma may be seen (fig. 26). The larger cells often have abundant clear cytoplasm with sharply outlined cell membranes (fig. 27). These typically contain abundant glycogen deposits. Other nodules may be composed of small cells with scanty eosinophilic cytoplasm.

The nuclei of adenoma cells are generally round and centrally placed (figs. 24, 25). The chromatin is dense and occasionally, small nucleoli are evident. Multinucleate adenoma cells may be prominent in some cases. As in other benign endocrine tumors enlarged, hyperchromatic nuclei may be evident in up to 25 percent of all adenomas (figs. 28, 29). Individual nuclei in such instances may measure up to 50 μm in diameter. Cells with enlarged hyperchromatic nuclei may be dispersed throughout the tumor or may be evident in small foci (9,17,43). In the

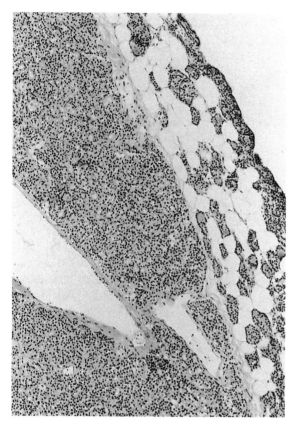

Figure 19
PARATHYROID ADENOMA
The rim contains numerous stromal fat cells.

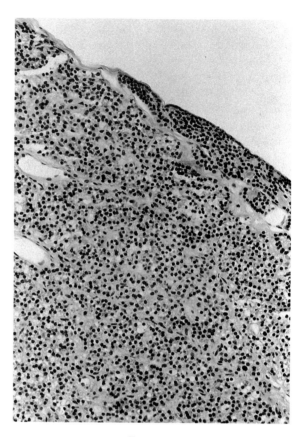

Figure 20
PARATHYROID ADENOMA
The rim is compressed and contains no stromal fat cells.

Figure 21
INTRATHYMIC
PARATHYROID
ADENOMA
Thymic tissue with a Hassal corpuscle at lower right. There is no rim of adjacent parathyroid in this portion of the adenoma.

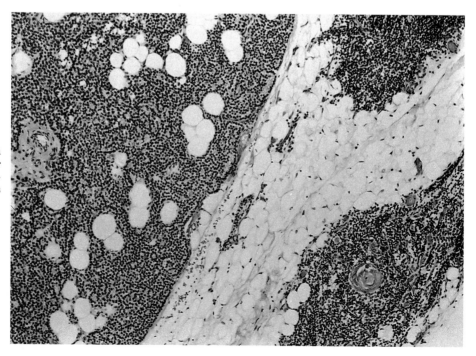

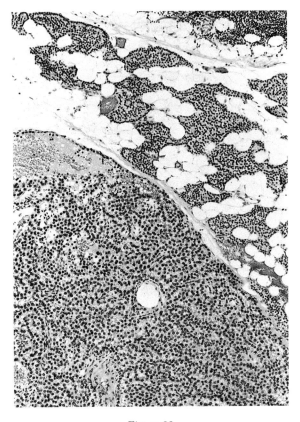

Figure 22
INTRATHYMIC PARATHYROID ADENOMA
In this same case as figure 18, a rim of normocellular parathyroid is present in this portion of the adenoma (X300).

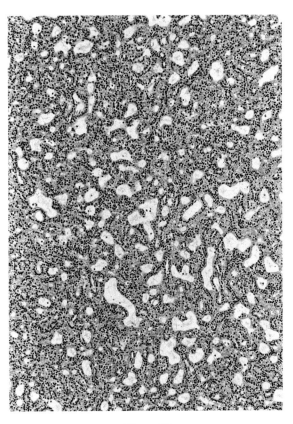

Figure 23
PARATHYROID ADENOMA
This tumor shows a glandular (tubular) pattern throughout.

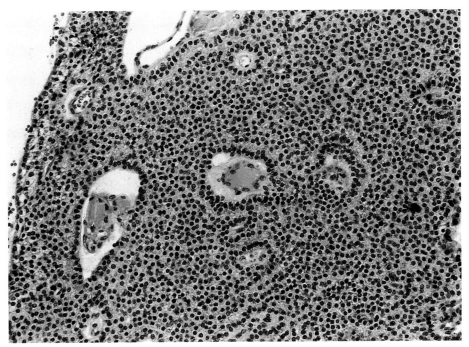

Figure 24
PARATHYROID
ADENOMA
The tumor cells have a palisaded arrangement around blood vessels.

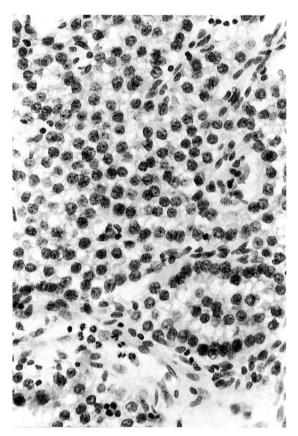

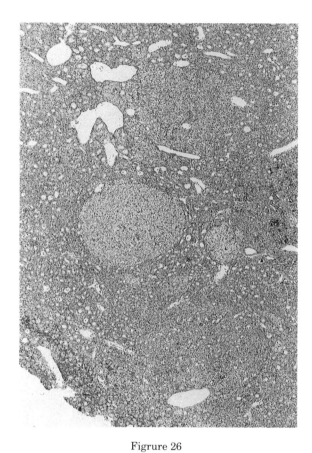

Figure 25
PARATHYROID ADENOMA
Monomorphic tumor cells with centrally placed hyperchromatic nuclei.

Figrrure 26
PARATHYROID ADENOMA
This tumor shows multiple ill-defined nodules in many areas. (Figures 26 and 27 are from the same patient.)

Figure 27
PARATHYROID
ADENOMA
Cells within the nodule have abundant clear cyto-plasm.

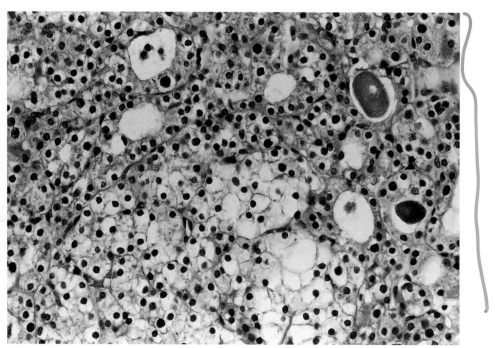

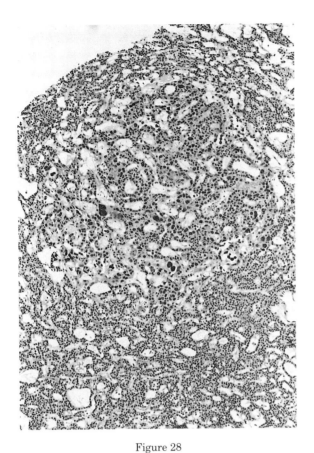

Figure 28
PARATHYROID ADENOMA
This section contains cells with enlarged hyperchromatic nuclei.

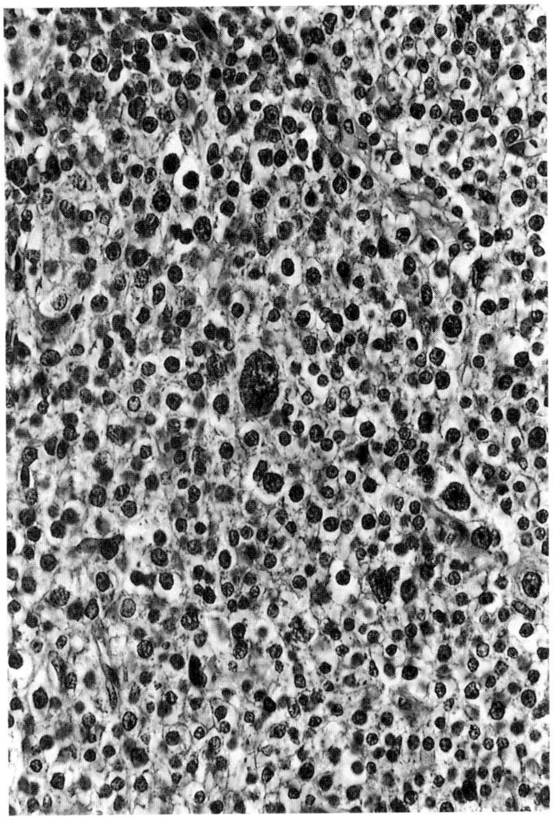

Figure 29
PARATHYROID ADENOMA
Cells with enlarged hyperchromatic nuclei are scattered throughout the tumor.

absence of other features of malignancy, the presence of hyperchromatic nuclei should not be used as a criterion for carcinoma. In fact, the presence of such bizarre nuclei may be used as a point in favor of the diagnosis of adenoma rather than carcinoma. Cells with enlarged hyperchromatic nuclei may be seen in fine-needle aspiration biopsy specimens of parathyroid adenomas (pl. VII).

The presence of a rim of normal or suppressed parathyroid tissue has been suggested as an important criterion to distinguish adenoma from hyperplasia (figs. 19, 20). The cells within the rim are typically smaller than those in the adenoma and contain more abundant parenchymal fat (pl. VIII). Generally, the fat droplets within the suppressed chief cells measure 0.5 to 1.5 mm in diameter (14,57). If fat is present within adenoma cells, it tends to be more finely dispersed than in the suppressed glands. Approximately 50 to 60

percent of cases reported as adenoma have a rim of non-neoplastic chief cells; generally, the probability of finding a rim is highest in small adenomas (see figs. 19, 20). Castleman and Mallory (16) reported that the probability of demonstrating a small fragment of parathyroid gland in or on the capsule of a tumor diminishes rapidly as the size of the tumor increases. They further stated that "partial or total atrophy" of the normal remnant is likely with large tumors.

Although the rim of the parathyroid is generally separated from the adenoma by a connective tissue capsule, the capsule may be indistinct or even absent in some cases.

Adenomas frequently contain cystic structures that are often surrounded by chief cells arranged in a cuboidal pattern (figs. 30, 31). The cysts may appear empty, but more commonly are filled with a PAS-positive eosinophilic homogeneous material

PLATE VII

PARATHYROID ADENOMA

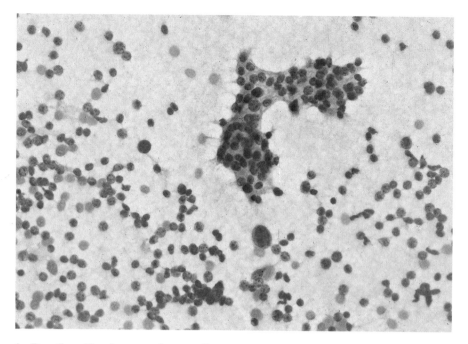

A. Parathyroid adenoma, fine-needle aspirate. Many of the nuclei are "naked." Clusters of cells with eosinophilic cytoplasm are also evident.

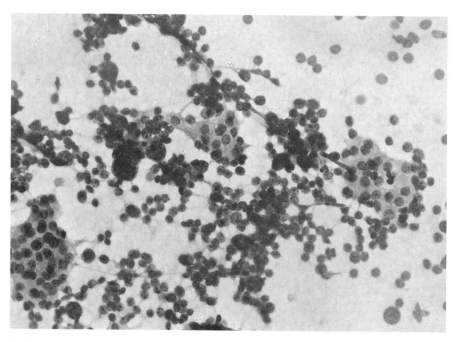

B. Parathyroid adenoma, fine-needle aspirate. Occasional cells with enlarged hyperchromatic nuclei are evident.

PLATE VIII

PARATHYROID ADENOMA

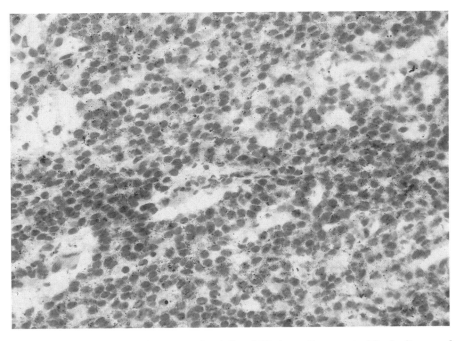

A. Parathyroid adenoma, frozen section (oil red O). A small amount of finely dispersed fat is present within the adenoma cells.

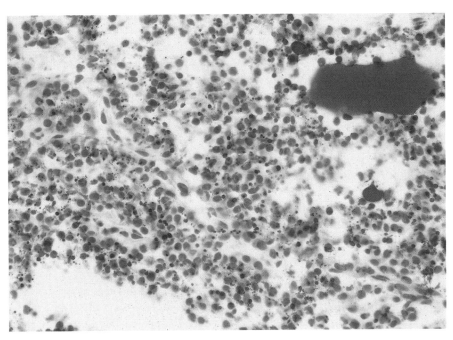

B. Parathyroid adenoma rim, frozen section (oil red O). The cells within the rim contain larger and more abundant lipid deposits than the adenoma cells.

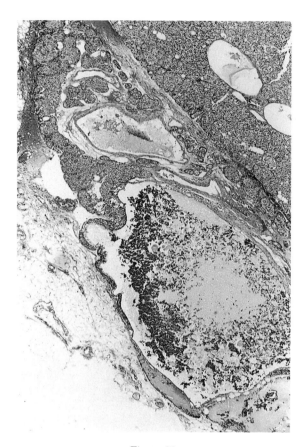

Figure 30
PARATHYROID ADENOMA
A focus of cystic change is present.

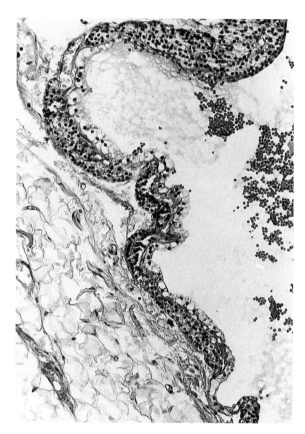

Figure 31
PARATHYROID ADENOMA
Many of the cells lining the cyst have a clear cytoplasm.

which shows a retraction-like artefact at its edges. This material bears a striking resemblance to thyroid colloid. Immunohistochemical studies, however, have revealed that the eosinophilic material is negative for thyroglobulin.

Scattered follicle-like or glandular structures may be identified in many adenomas. Some parathyroid adenomas, however, have an entirely follicular or tubular structure (see fig. 23). The eosinophilic material within the lumina is often concentrically laminated and may be focally calcified. Such intraluminal secretions may, therefore, resemble psammoma bodies. Congo red stains reveal that some of the eosinophilic intraluminal material shows green birefringence typical of amyloid (7). Sometimes cellular debris is present within the follicles, and the studies of Boquist (15) suggest that these follicles arise as a result of degenerative changes within the epithelium of hyperfunctioning parathyroid tissue.

The formation of papillae rarely occurs in parathyroid adenomas (26). In a review of 103 adenomas, Sahin and Robinson (61) identified a single case in which the tumor had a partially papillary architecture. The papillae were formed of fibrovascular cores which were covered by cells with abundant eosinophilic cytoplasm and round nuclei with punctate chromatin. The tumor did not contain psammoma bodies and immunoperoxidase stains for thyroglobulin were negative. Rarely, fine-needle aspiration biopsy leads to a mistaken diagnosis of papillary carcinoma of the thyroid in patients with parathyroid adenomas (26).

Parathyroid microadenomas may be impossible to differentiate from focally hyperplastic glands since the lesions are usually not encapsulated (4). However, other parathyroid glands removed from patients with microadenomas have proven to be normocellular. Moreover, surgical removal of the microadenomas has resulted in normalization of serum calcium levels (39,53).

Most descriptions of parathyroid adenomas stress the absence of stromal fat as a major criterion for distinguishing adenoma from hyperplasia (13). However, careful study reveals that adenomas may contain at least some stromal fat cells. These may be distributed uniformly throughout the adenoma or may be present in small aggregates. Sometimes, the fat may be so abundant that a small biopsy is interpreted as a normocellular gland. The presence of fat, therefore, within the stroma of an enlarged parathyroid gland does not exclude the diagnosis of adenoma.

The stroma of adenomas contains abundant capillaries which can be demonstrated selectively using antibodies to the factor VIII–related antigen or *Ulex europaeus*. Adenoma cells may be arranged around the blood vessels in a pseudorosette-like pattern (fig. 24); some adenomas exhibit pronounced stromal edema (figs. 32, 33).

The stroma of adenomas is generally sparse. Occasionally, however, adenomas contain considerable amounts of fibrous connective tissue, and there is rarely focal deposition of amyloid. The fibrous bands may be similar to those seen in cases of parathyroid carcinoma. Fibrosis most likely develops because of degenerative changes within the adenoma, and the fibrotic areas frequently show hemosiderin deposition and chronic inflammation. Cystic degeneration of an adenoma may lead to considerable capsular fibrosis (fig. 34). Areas of capsular and intratumoral fibrosis may be extensively calcified and even ossified.

The presence of mitoses is generally regarded as a criterion of malignancy in parathyroid neoplasms. However, several studies indicate that mitotic activity may be present in benign lesions of the parathyroid, including adenomas and hyperplasias (pl. IX–A). Snover and Foucar (63) found parenchymal mitoses in 71 percent of adenomas. In this series, the number of mitoses was averaged for the entire section examined with 80 to 160 high-power fields examined per case. Fifty-nine percent of their cases contained less than 1 mitosis per 10 high-power fields, while 12 percent had more than 1 mitosis per 10 high-power fields. None of the patients had evidence of recurrent or metastatic disease with a median follow-up of 5.5 years.

In a series of 92 cases reviewed by San-Juan et al. (62), mitoses were identified in 39 (42 percent); 13 (14 percent) had more than 1 mitosis per 10 high-power fields. Three of 19 cases (16 percent) with mitoses and 1 of 7 cases (14 percent) without mitoses recurred. A single case with more than 1 mitosis per 10 high-power fields which recurred after initial surgery was considered a carcinoma. These data indicate that occasional mitotic activity may be present in adenomas and that mitotic activity by itself cannot be considered a criterion of malignancy. Cases with more than 1 mitosis per 10 high-power fields, however, should be evaluated carefully for the presence of other criteria suggestive of carcinoma.

Immunohistochemistry and Flow Cytometry. The immunohistochemical features of normal parathyroid glands are discussed in the chapter on The Normal Parathyroid. Generally, neoplastic chief cells contain the low molecular weight cytokeratins 8 (52 kD), 18 (45 kD), and 19 (40 kD). In addition, neurofilament proteins have been demonstrated in some cases. Chromogranin A (parathyroid secretory protein I) is also present within most normal and neoplastic chief cells. Although parathyroid hormone has been demonstrated within adenomas by immunohistochemistry (50), the demonstration of parathyroid hormone mRNA by in situ hybridization appears to provide more consistent results (pl. IX–B) (35,64).

Flow cytometric studies have demonstrated that most adenomas have a significant component of tetraploid cells (44). However, different authors have used different "cutoff" values to assign a case to the tetraploid group. Aneuploidy has been demonstrated in 3 to 25 percent of adenomas (44).

Ultrastructural Findings. The studies of Roth and Munger (58) indicate that the cells comprising most parathyroid adenomas have lost the normal integrated secretory and synthetic functions typical of normal chief cells. Often, it is impossible to determine whether individual cells are in resting or synthetic phases of their cycles (18).

It should also be noted that individual adenoma cells do not necessarily have higher endocrine activities than cells in the adjacent rim. Enhanced secretory activity is largely a function of the increased total mass of a parathyroid adenoma, although occasional cells within an adenoma may show very strong signals for parathyroid hormone messenger RNA (mRNA) (35). This conclusion is supported, in part, on the basis of in

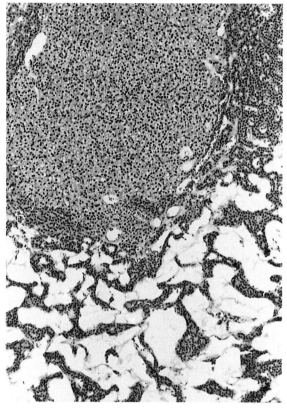

Figure 32
PARATHYROID ADENOMA
The stroma is markedly edematous with abundant fat. A nodule within the adenoma is composed of transitional oncocytic cells. (Figures 32 and 33 are from the same patient.)

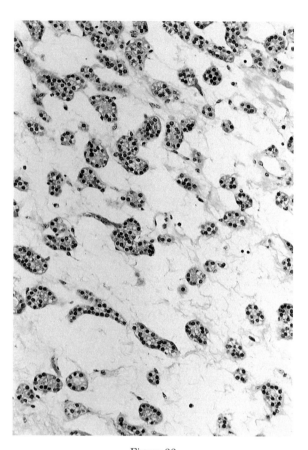

Figure 33
PARATHYROID ADENOMA
The cells embedded within the edematous stroma are vacuolated chief cells.

Figure 34
PARATHYROID
ADENOMA
This adenoma shows extensive cystic change. The wall is fibrotic and contains entrapped chief cells.

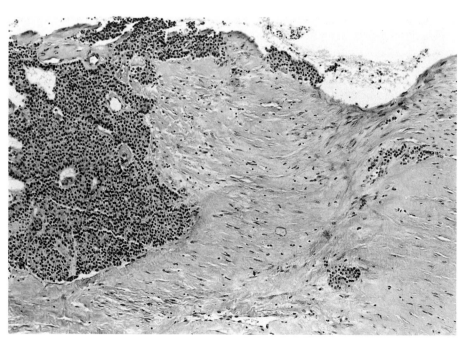

PLATE IX

PARATHYROID ADENOMA

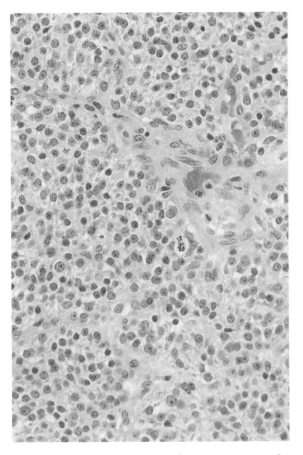

A. This parathyroid adenoma has an average of 1 mitosis per 10 high-power fields.

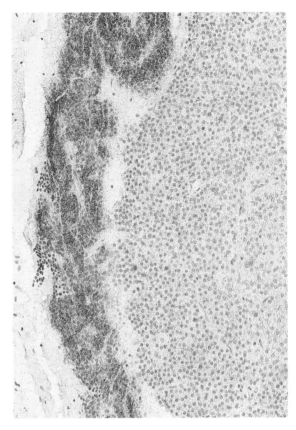

B. Autoradiograph, in situ hybridization using a 35-S–labeled antisense RNA probe for pre-pro-parathyroid hormone mRNA. The cells of the rim show an intense hybridization signal, while the cells in the adenoma show much less label. (Courtesy of Dr. Hubert J. Wolfe, Boston, MA.)

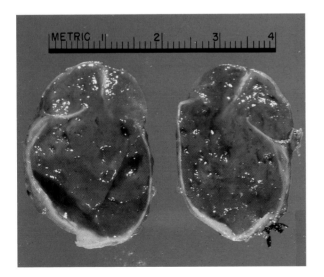

C. In this oncocytic type of parathyroid adenoma, the tumor is red-brown on cross section.

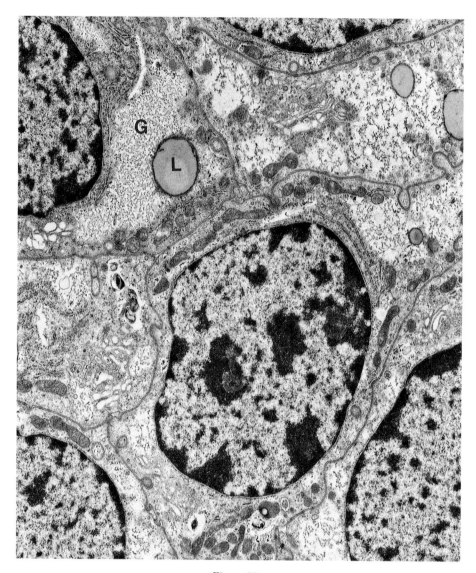

Figure 35
PARATHYROID ADENOMA
Electron micrograph of parathyroid adenoma. The cells show interdigitated plasma membranes, occasional lipid droplets (L), glycogen (G), and very few secretory granules (X13,200).

situ hybridization studies using antisense probes to parathyroid mRNA (64). Adenoma cells may show less parathyroid mRNA than the cells within the uninvolved rim of the gland (pl. IX–B).

The plasma membranes of adenoma cells frequently show more complex interdigitations than do normal chief cells (figs. 35, 36). Moreover, adenomas are more likely to show greater degrees of mitochondrial pleomorphism. Generally, adenomas have more extensive endoplasmic reticulum and larger Golgi regions with increased numbers

of vesicles as compared to normal or suppressed chief cells. There are no apparent increases in the numbers of prosecretory granules or mature secretory granules, although lysosomes may be more prominent (18,58).

Aguillar-Parada and co-workers (2) have described in detail the ultrastructural features of a parathyroid adenoma associated with severe hypercalcemia. The cells were characterized by the presence of numerous microvilli, abundant rough surfaced endoplasmic reticulum, prominent

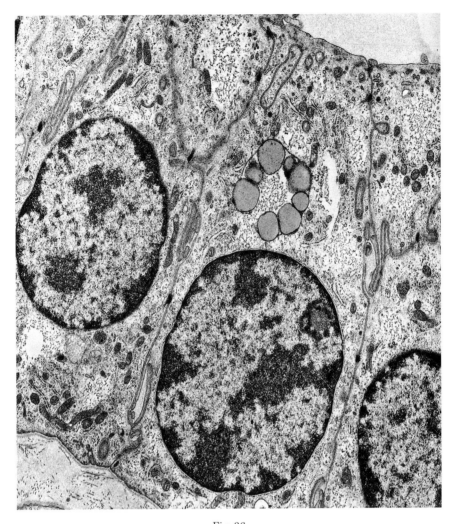

Fig. 36
PARATHYROID ADENOMA
In this electron micrograph the tumor cells are arranged in glandular formations. Plasma membranes show complex interdigitations. There are very few secretory granules. Supranuclear lipid droplets are evident in some cells (X12,980).

nuclear pores, and annulate lamellae. Adenomas with lesser degrees of hypercalcemia did not have these features, and Aguillar-Parada suggested that surface microvilli formation correlated with the degree of synthetic activity within the tumor cells.

Adenoma Variants. *Oncocytic adenomas* of the parathyroid gland are uncommon, and some authors have considered them to be nonfunctional neoplasms. It should be remembered that oncocytic cells increase in number with age, and that some of the cells form large nodular aggregates or oncocytic nodules. Such nodules are common in the parathyroids of elderly individuals and are not generally considered to represent

adenomas by most authors. However, this distinction may be difficult.

Recent studies, however, indicate that hyperparathyroidism may be associated with oncocytic parathyroid adenomas (46,50,52,69). In a review of 160 parathyroid adenomas, Bedetti (10) found 10 (6.25 percent) that were composed exclusively or predominantly of oncocytic cells. The tumors had an average weight of 1.2 g.

In cases reported by Wolpert and co-workers (69), oncocytic adenomas accounted for 3 percent of all parathyroid adenomas. The major criteria for the diagnosis of oncocytic parathyroid adenoma, according to these authors, include: 1) at

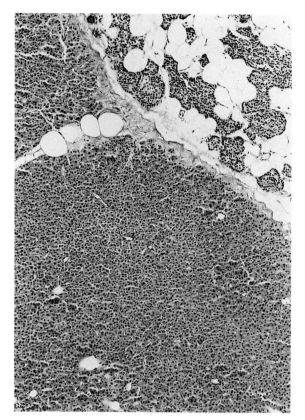

Figure 37
PARATHYROID ADENOMA,
ONCOCYTIC TYPE

A rim of normal parathyroid is present in the left upper portion of the field.

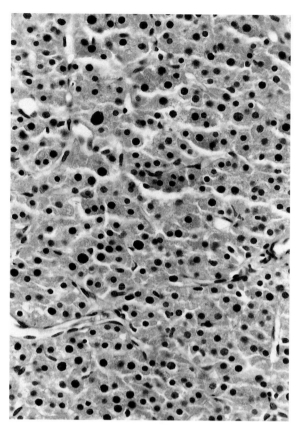

Figure 38
PARATHYROID ADENOMA,
ONCOCYTIC TYPE

The cells have round hyperchromatic nuclei and abundant granular cytoplasm.

least 90 percent composition by oncocytic cells; 2) a second histologically normal parathyroid; and 3) postoperative alleviation of hypercalcemia. More than 50 percent of previously reported cases of oncocytic parathyroid adenoma, however, did not conform to these criteria (69).

On gross appearance, oncocytic adenomas are soft and range in color from tan or dark brown to orange (pl. IX–C). Most tumors are ellipsoidal or spherical, and they may be smooth, lobulated, or nodular. In Wolpert's series, the adenomas had a median weight of 2.8 g and a median diameter of 2.5 cm.

The cells are arranged in broad sheets, anastomosing cords, or in acinar patterns (figs. 37, 38). The oncocytic cells have abundant granular eosinophilic cytoplasm and nuclei which are round with dense chromatin. Some exhibit considerable variation in nuclear size with occasional bizarre hyperchromatic forms. Occasionally, groups of

multinucleate cells, similar to those found in chief cell adenomas, are also present.

In 8 of the 15 cases reported by Wolpert (69), a rim of normal parathyroid was present adjacent to the adenoma. Similar to chief cell adenomas, the cells of the oncocytic adenomas had less parenchymal fat as compared to the cells in the rims of the normal parathyroid.

Ultrastructural studies have revealed that oncocytic cells are filled with mitochondria (fig. 39). The cells typically contain abundant cytochrome c oxidase, and secretory and prosecretory granules are present in relatively low numbers.

While earlier studies indicated that oncocytic cells were nonfunctional, immunohistochemical analyses using antibodies to parathyroid hormone revealed immunoreactive hormone within these cells. Moreover, in situ hybridization analyses revealed relatively abundant parathyroid

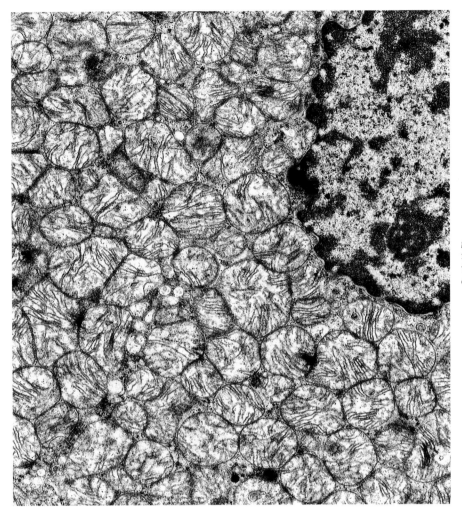

Figure 39
PARATHYROID
ADENOMA,
ONCOCYTIC TYPE
In this electron micrograph of parathyroid adenoma, oncocytic type, the cytoplasm is filled with mitochondria (X16,000).

mRNA within some oncocytic cells (64). These data support the view that oncocytic cells may be functional and that functional oncocytic parathyroid adenomas do, indeed, exist.

Lipoadenomas (hamartomas) are rare benign neoplasms characterized by the proliferation of parenchymal and stromal elements (1,28,37,67). These tumors are also referred to as hamartomas (49). They are usually associated with hyperparathyroidism.

The typical lipoadenoma presents as an encapsulated mass which appears soft, yellow-tan, and lobulated on cross section (fig. 40). The tumors weigh between 0.5 and 420 g. Occasionally, chief cell adenomas exhibit small foci of lipoadenomatous change.

The stroma of lipoadenomas is characterized by an abundance of adipose tissue showing frequent areas of myxoid change and fibrosis (figs. 41–43). Prominent collections of lymphoid cells are seen in some cases. The parenchymal elements of lipoadenomas include chief cells and small numbers of oncocytic cells arranged in a thin, branching, cord-like fashion (figs. 41–43).

Lipoadenomas have also been reported in the neck and mediastinum, and all of the published cases have been benign.

Adenoma-Associated Parathyroid Glands.
Classically, nonadenomatous glands from patients with parathyroid adenoma have been described as having lower glandular and parenchymal weights and greater amounts of stromal fat than parathyroids from normocalcemic individuals (fig. 44). In most instances, however, adenoma-associated parathyroid glands are indistinguishable from glands of normocalcemic individuals

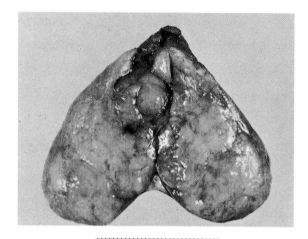

Figure 40
PARATHYROID LIPOADENOMA
The cross section shows an encapsulated tumor with a lobular pattern. (Fig. 50 from Fascicle 14, Second Series.)

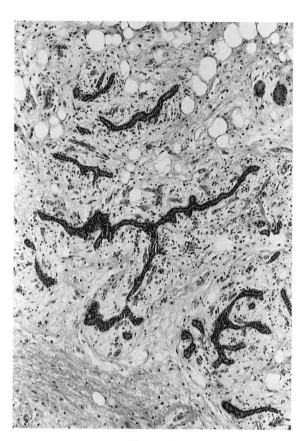

Figure 42
PARATHYROID LIPOADENOMA
The chief cells are arranged in branching narrow cords.

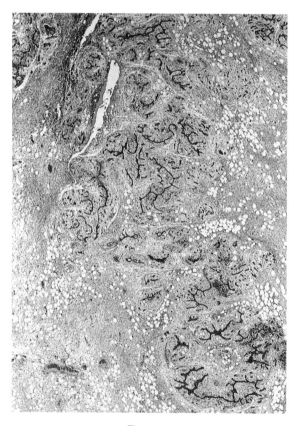

Figure 41
PARATHYROID LIPOADENOMA
The tumor shows a distinctive lobular pattern. The stroma contains both fat and fibrous tissue.

using standard histopathologic criteria. Generally, adenoma-associated parathyroid glands contain abundant fat within the parenchymal cells which is independent of the stromal fat content (57).

Ultrastructural analyses reveal reduced complexity and interdigitations of plasma membranes, reduction in the amount of granular endoplasmic reticulum and Golgi regions, smaller numbers of secretory granules and prosecretory granules, and increased amounts of cytoplasmic lipid (23).

Differential Diagnosis. Parathyroid adenomas must be distinguished from carcinomas and from hyperplasias of the parathyroid glands, as discussed on pp. 58 and 76. The diagnosis of parathyroid adenoma and its distinction from other neoplasms occurring in this region is usually straightforward, since most patients have evidence of associated hypercalcemia together with increased parathyroid hormone levels. Sometimes, however, it is difficult to distinguish

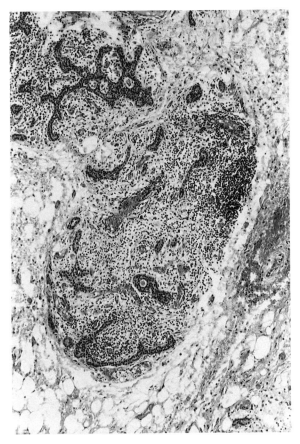

Figure 43
PARATHYROID LIPOADENOMA
Focal aggregates of lymphocytes are present in this lobule of tumor.

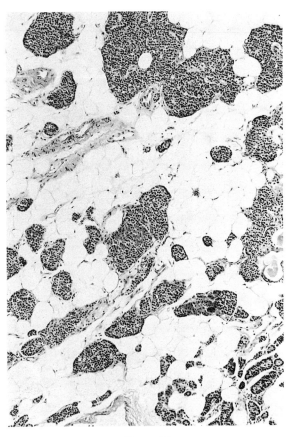

Figure 44
NORMAL PARATHYROID
FROM PATIENT WITH ADENOMA
The ratio of parenchymal cells to fat cells is very low in this case.

primary thyroid neoplasms of both follicular and C-cell type from parathyroid adenomas. Since approximately 0.2 percent of normal parathyroids lie within the thyroid parenchyma and a significant proportion lie within the capsule of the gland, parathyroid adenomas may have the gross appearance of a primary thyroid tumor (41).

Parathyroid adenomas with a completely follicular or acinar pattern of growth are rare, but foci of follicular change are relatively common. In this situation, deeper sections will often reveal areas more typical of parathyroid with solid cell sheets or cells showing a cord-like pattern of growth.

Occasionally, thyroid adenomas contain abundant stromal fat cells and are classified as lipoadenomas (21,30). These lesions, particularly when there is a microfollicular growth pattern, are especially difficult to distinguish from parathyroid adenomas and hyperplasias. Generally, however,

the cells of parathyroid adenomas and hyperplasias appear smaller and more vacuolated than cells comprising thyroid follicular adenomas. Moreover, the nuclei of parathyroid cells are generally rounder and have a denser chromatin pattern than the nuclei of thyroid follicular epithelium. LiVolsi (41) noted that in contrast to primary thyroid clear cell tumors, parathyroid adenomas occurring within the thyroid have a more delicate vascular pattern.

Parathyroid adenomas contain more glycogen than do tumors of thyroid follicular origin, and the PAS stain is particularly helpful in this situation. Diastase-resistant PAS-positive material in thyroid follicular epithelium usually represents colloid or lipofuscin. Most thyroid follicular epithelial neoplasms contain little glycogen, except for the occasional clear cell types which contain more abundant glycogen deposits.

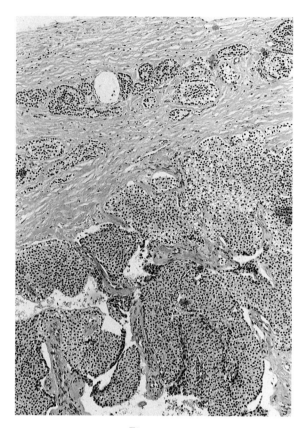

Figure 45
ATYPICAL PARATHYROID ADENOMA
Groups of neoplastic chief cells are entrapped within the thickened fibrous capsule. (Figures 45 and 46 are from the same patient.)

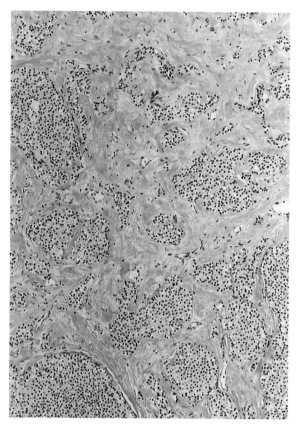

Figure 46
ATYPICAL PARATHYROID ADENOMA
The central region of the tumor shows considerable fibrosis.

Immunohistochemistry is of particular importance in distinguishing thyroid from parathyroid tumors. Thyroid follicular tumors typically show thyroglobulin positivity both within the tumor cells and within the luminal colloid. Parathyroid adenomas, including those with a follicular pattern, are negative for thyroglobulin. Chromogranin immunoreactivity is usually present in parathyroid tumors, while thyroid follicular epithelium is negative (68). Antibodies to parathyroid hormone (50) or nucleic acid probes for parathyroid hormone mRNA (35,64) are also useful for the positive identification of parathyroid tissue.

Parathyroid adenomas rarely contain papillary structures (26). The presence of finely granular chromatin with nuclear pseudoinclusions, together with thyroglobulin positivity, distinguishes thyroid papillary carcinoma from papillary formations in parathyroid adenomas.

Similarly, oncocytic parathyroid tumors are negative for thyroglobulin, whereas oncocytic thyroid follicular neoplasms are usually thyroglobulin positive.

Some parathyroid adenomas are difficult to distinguish from medullary thyroid carcinomas. Most medullary carcinomas have a finely granular eosinophilic cytoplasm, although some have a clear cytoplasm. The nuclei of medullary carcinoma cells are larger and more vesicular than those of parathyroid tumor cells. Moreover, medullary carcinomas are usually positive for calcitonin, chromogranin, and carcinoembryonic antigen, whereas parathyroid adenomas are positive only for chromogranin (20).

Parathyroid adenomas may show some of the features associated with parathyroid carcinomas (figs. 45, 46). These include adherence of the tumor to the adjacent soft tissues, mitotic activity, trabecular growth pattern, capsular invasion, and the presence of broad fibrous bands. The term *atypical adenoma* is used to describe neoplasms that have some of these features but lack unequivocal evidence of malignancy, such as soft tissue and vascular invasion (38). A diagnosis of atypical adenoma implies that the behavior of the neoplasm is unpredictable with respect to recurrence and metastasis.

Static DNA fluorometric methods have been used to a limited extent to characterize atypical adenomas. Levin (38) reported aneuploidy in 4 of 9 parathyroid carcinomas, including 2 cases that had been classified initially as atypical adenomas. Both of these patients developed recurrent disease and 1 died of hepatic metastases. None of the 10 patients with a final diagnosis of atypical adenoma (nonaneuploid) has had evidence of recurrence with an average follow-up of 25 months. These findings suggest that the demonstration of aneuploidy by static DNA fluorometric methods in lesions diagnosed as atypical adenomas should lead to close patient follow-up to rule out recurrence or metastasis (38). The significance of the demonstration of aneuploidy by flow cytometric methods is considerably less clear (44), as discussed on p. 97.

Prognosis and Treatment. The treatment of patients with parathyroid adenoma has been controversial (32). While some surgeons favor subtotal parathyroidectomy in all patients with hyper-parathyroidism (including those with adenoma) (51), most other surgeons employ a more conservative approach, with excision of the adenoma and biopsy of at least one additional normal sized gland (48).

Rudberg and co-workers (59) reported recurrent hypercalcemia in only 3 percent (10 of 339) of patients with a diagnosis of adenoma who were treated conservatively, i.e. excision of the single enlarged gland; recurrent hypercalcemia did not develop earlier than 9 years after the initial surgery. New adenomas were identified in two patients who had surgical re-exploration of the neck.

Recurrence of hypercalcemia following excision of parathyroid adenoma may also occur as a result of inadvertent implantation of parathyroid tissue during surgery (24). Foci of implanted parathyroid tissue are generally associated with considerable fibrosis with adherence to the adjacent normal tissues. Such cases may be extremely difficult to differentiate histologically from parathyroid carcinoma. Implantation of parathyroid tissue is most likely to occur if the capsule of the adenoma has been transgressed during surgery (24,55).

REFERENCES

1. Abul-Haj SK, Conklin H, Hewitt WC. Functioning lipoadenoma of the parathyroid gland: report of a unique case. N Engl J Med 1962;266:121–23.
2. Aguillar-Parada E, González-Angulo A, Del Peön L, Mravko E. Functioning microvillous adenoma of the parathyroid gland containing nuclear pores and annulate lamellae. Hum Pathol 1985;16:511–16.
3. Akerström G, Bergström R, Grimelius L, et al. Relation between changes in clinical and histopathological features of primary hyperparathyroidism. World J Surg 1986;10:696–702.
4. _____, Rudberg C, Grimelius L et al. Histologic parathyroid abnormalities in an autopsy series. Hum Pathol 1986;17:520–27.
5. Allo MD, Thompson NW. Familial hyperparathyroidism caused by solitary adenomas. Surgery 1982;92:486–90.
6. Altenähr E, Arps H, Montz R, Dorn G. Quantitative ultrastructural and radioimmunologic assessment of parathyroid gland activity in primary hyperparathyroidism. Lab Invest 1979;41:303–12.
7. Anderson TJ, Ewen SW. Amyloid in normal and pathological parathyroid glands. J Clin Pathol 1974;27:656–63.
8. Arnold A, Staunton CE, Kim HG, Gaz RD, Kronenberg HM. Monoclonality and abnormal parathyroid hormone genes in parathyroid adenomas. N Engl J Med 1988;318:658–62.
9. Banerjee SS, Faragher B, Hasleton PS. Nuclear diameter in parathyroid disease. J Clin Pathol 1983;36:143–48.
10. Bedetti CD, Dekker A, Watson CG. Functioning oxyphil cell adenoma of the parathyroid gland. A clinicopathologic study of ten patients with hyperparathyroidism. Hum Pathol 1984;15:1121–6.
11. Black WC. Correlative light and electron microscopy in primary hyperparathyroidism. Arch Pathol 1969;88:225-41.
12. Black BK, Ackerman LV. Tumors of the parathyroid. A review of 23 cases. Cancer 1950;3:415–44.
13. Black WC, Utley JR. The differential diagnosis of parathyroid adenoma and chief cell hyperplasia. Am J Clin Pathol 1968;49:761–75.
14. Bondeson AG, Bondeson L, Ljungberg O, Tibblin S. Fat staining in parathyroid disease—diagnostic value and impact on surgical strategy: Clinicopathologic analysis of 191 cases. Hum Pathol 1985;16:1255–63.
15. Boquist, L. Follicles in human parathyroid glands. Lab Invest 1973;28:313–20.
16. Castleman B, Mallory TB. The pathology of the parathyroid gland in hyperparathyroidism—a study of 25 cases. Am J Pathol 1935;11:1–72.
17. _____, Roth SI. Tumors of the parathyroid glands. Atlas of Tumor Pathology, 2nd Series, Fascicle 14. Washington, D.C.: Armed Forces Institute of Pathology, 1978, 1–94.
18. Cinti S, Colussi G, Minola E, Dickersin GR. Parathyroid glands in primary hyperparathyroidism: an ultrastructural study of 50 cases. Hum Pathol 1986;17:1036–46.
19. Cohn KH, Silen W. Lessons of parathyroid reoperations. Am J Surg 1982;144:511–7.
20. DeLellis RA, Wolfe HJ. The pathobiology of the human calcitonin C-cell: a review. Pathol Annu 1981;16:25–52.
21. DeRienzo D, Truong L. Thyroid neoplasms containing mature fat: a report of two cases and review of the literature. Mod Pathol 1989;2:506–10.
22. Edis AJ. Surgical anatomy and technique of neck exploration for primary hyperparathyroidism. Surg Clin North Am 1977;57:495–504.
23. Ejerblad S, Grimelius L, Johansson H, Werner I. Studies on the non-adenomatous glands in patients with a solitary parathyroid adenoma. Ups J Med Sci 1976;81:31–6.
24. Fraker DL, Travis WD, Merendino JJ Jr, et al. Locally recurrent parathyroid neoplasms as a cause for recurrent and persistent primary hyperparathyroidism. Ann Surg 1991;213:58–65.
25. Friedman E, Sakaguchi K, Bale AE, et al. Clonality of parathyroid tumors in familial multiple endocrine neoplasia type I. N Engl J Med 1989;321:1057
26. Friedman M, Shimaoka K, Lopez AC, Shedd DP. Parathyroid adenoma diagnosed as papillary carcinoma of the thyroid on needle aspiration smears. Acta Cytol 1983;27:337–40.
27. Gagel RF, Tashjian AH Jr, Cummings T, et al. The clinical outcome of prospective screening for multiple endocrine neoplasia type 2a: an 18 year experience. N Engl J Med 1988;318:478–84.
28. Geelhoed GW. Parathyroid adenolipoma: clinical and morphological features. Surgery 1982;92:806–10.
29. Ghandur-Mnaymneh L, Kimura N. The parathyroid adenoma. A histopathologic definition with a study of 172 cases of primary hyperparathyroidism. Am J Pathol 1984;115:70–83.
30. Gnepp DR, Ogorzalek JM, Heffess CS. Fat-containing lesions of the thyroid gland. Am J Surg Pathol 1989;13:605–12.
31. Golden A, Canary JJ, Kerwin DM. Concurrence of hyperplasia and neoplasia of the parathyroid glands. Am J Med 1965;38:562–78.
32. Goldman L, Gordau GS, Roof BS. The parathyroids: progress, problems and practice. Curr Probl Surg 1971;8:1–64.
33. Harness JK, Ramsburg SR, Nishiyama RH, Thompson NW. Multiple adenomas of the parathyroids: do they exist? Arch Surg 1979;114:468–74.
34. Jackson CE, Cerny JC, Block MA, Fialkow PJ. Probable clonal origin of aldosteronomas versus multicellular origin of parathyroid adenomas. Surgery 1982;92:875–9.
35. Kendall CH, Roberts PA, Pringle JL, Lauder I. The expression of parathyroid hormone messenger RNA in normal and abnormal parathyroid tissue. J Pathol 1991;165:111–8.
36. Kramer WM. Association of parathyroid hyperplasia with neoplasia. Am J Clin Pathol 1970;53:275–83.
37. LeGolvan DP, Moore BP, Nishiyama RH. Parathyroid hamartoma. Report of two cases and review of the literature. Am J Clin Pathol 1977;67:31–5.
38. Levin KE, Chew KL, Ljung BM, et al. Deoxyribonucleic acid cytometry helps identify parathyroid carcinomas. J Clin Endocrinol Metab 1988;67:779–84.
39. Liechty RD, Teter A, Suba EJ. The tiny parathyroid adenoma. Surgery 1986;100:1048–52.
40. Lips CJ, Vasen HF, Lamers CB. Multiple endocrine neoplasia syndromes. CRC Critical Rev Oncol Hematol 1984;2:117-24.

41. LiVolsi VA. Surgical pathology of the thyroid gland. Philadelphia: WB Saunders, 1990.

42. LiVolsi LA, LoGerfo P, Feind CR. Coexistent parathyroid adenomas and thyroid carcinomas. Can radiation be blamed? Arch Surg 1978;113:285-6.

43. Lloyd HM, Jacobi JM, Cooke RA. Nuclear diameter in parathyroid adenomas. J Clin Pathol 1979;32:1278-81.

44. Mallette LE. DNA quantitation in the study of parathyroid lesions. A review. Am J Clin Pathol 1992;98:305–11.

45. Marx SJ. Genetic defects in primary hyperparathyroidism [Editorial]. N Engl J Med 1988;318:699-701.

46. McGregor DH, Lotuaco LG, Rao MS, Chu LL. Functioning oxyphil adenoma of parathyroid gland. An ultrastructural and biochemical study. Am J Pathol 1978;92:691-711.

47. Nishiyama R, Farhi D, Thompson NW. Radiation exposure and the simultaneous occurrence of primary hyperparathyroidism and thyroid nodules. Surg Clin North Am 1979;59:65-75.

48. Norton JA, Aurbach GD, Marx SJ, Doppman JL. Surgical management of hyperparathyroidism. In: DeGroot LJ, ed. Endocrinology, Vol. 2. 2nd ed. Philadelphia: WB Saunders 1989:1013-31.

49. Ober WB, Kaiser GA. Hamartoma of the parathyroid. Cancer 1958;11:601-6.

50. Ordonez NG, Ibanez ML, Mackay B, et al. Functioning oxyphil cell adenomas of parathyroid gland: immunoperoxidase evidence of hormonal activity in oxyphil cells. Am J Clin Pathol 1982;78:681-9.

51. Paloyan E, Lawrence AM, Baker WH, Straus FH II. Near total parathyroidectomy. Surg Clin North Am 1969;49:43-8.

52. Poole GV Jr, Albertson DA, Marshall RB, Myers RT. Oxyphil cell adenomas and hyperparathyroidism. Surgery 1982;92:799-805.

53. Prinz RA, Barbato AL, Braithwaite SS, et al. Prior irradiation and the development of coexistent differentiated thyroid cancer and hyperparathyroidism. Cancer 1982;49:874-7.

54. Rasbach DA, Monchik JM, Geelhoed GW, Harrison TS. Solitary parathyroid microadenoma. Surgery 1984;96:1092-8.

55. Rattner DW, Marrone GC, Kasdon E, Silen W. Recurrent hyperparathyroidism due to implantation of parathyroid tissue. Am J Surg 1985;149:745-8.

56. Reiling RE, Cady B, Clerkin EP. Aberrant parathyroid adenoma within the vagus nerve. Lahey Clin Bull 1972;25:158-62.

57. Roth SI, Gallagher MJ. The rapid identification of "normal" parathyroid glands by the presence of intracellular fat. Am J Pathol 1976;84:521-8.

58. _____, Munger BL. The cytology of the adenomatous, atrophic and hyperplastic parathyroid glands of man. A light and electron-microscopic study. Virchows Arch [A] 1962;335:389-410.

59. Rudberg C, Akerström G, Palmer M, et al. Late results of operation for primary hyperparathyroidism in 441 patients. Surgery 1986;99:643-51.

60. Russ, JE, Scanlon EF, Sener SF. Parathyroid adenomas following irradiation. Cancer 1979;43:1078-83.

61. Sahin A, Robinson RA. Papillae formation in parathyroid adenoma. A source of possible diagnostic error. Arch Pathol Lab Med 1988;112:99-100.

62. San-Juan J, Monteagudo C, Fraker D, Norton J, Merino MJ. Significance of mitotic activity and other morphologic parameters in parathyroid adenomas and their correlation with clinical behavior [Abstract]. Am J Clin Pathol 1989;92:523.

63. Snover DC, Foucar K. Mitotic activity in benign parathyroid disease. Am J Clin Pathol 1981;75:345-7.

64. Stork PJ, Herteaux C, Frazier R, Kronenburg H, Wolfe HJ. Expression and distribution of parathyroid hormone and parathyroid messenger RNA in pathological conditions of the parathyroid [Abstract]. Lab Invest 1989;60:92A.

65. Tisell LE, Carlsson S, Lindberg S, Ragnhult I. Autonomous hyperparathyroidism: a possible late complication of neck radiotherapy. Acta Chir Scand 1976;142:367-73.

66. Verdonk CA, Edis AJ. Parathyroid "double adenomas": fact or fiction? Surgery 1981;90:523-6.

67. Weiland LH, Garrison RC, Remine WH, Scholz DA. Lipoadenoma of the parathyroid gland. Am J Surg Pathol 1978;2:3-7.

68. Wilson BS, Lloyd RV. Detection of chromogranin in neuroendocrine cells with a monoclonal antibody. Am J Pathol 1984;115:458-68.

69. Wolpert HR, Vickery AL Jr, Wang CA. Functioning oxyphil cell adenomas of the parathyroid gland. A study of 15 cases. Am J Surg Pathol 1989;13:500-4.

70. Woolner LB, Keating FR Jr, Black BM. Tumors and hyperplasia of the parathyroid glands—a review of the pathological findings in 140 cases of primary hyperparathyroidism. Cancer 1952;5:1069-88.

PARATHYROID CARCINOMA

Definition. A malignant tumor derived from the parenchymal cells of the parathyroid gland.

General Features. Parathyroid carcinoma is a rare neoplasm which accounts for 0.5 to 2 percent of cases of primary hyperparathyroidism (3,4,15). The tumor has a high probability of local recurrence and the potential, late in its course, to metastasize to regional nodes and distant sites (27).

Clinical Features. In contrast to adenomas, which occur more commonly in women, the sex ratio of patients with parathyroid carcinoma is approximately equal (23,27). In cases reported by Wang and Gaz (27), the age range was 28 to 72 years with a mean of 45 years.

Most patients have evidence of metabolic complications at presentation with marked symptomatic hypercalcemia. The serum calcium levels are typically in excess of 14 mg/dl with marked elevations of parathyroid hormone. Some patients with parathyroid carcinoma present with hypercalcemic crisis. In most cases, the degree of hypercalcemia is greater in patients with carcinoma than in those with adenoma. Occasionally, parathyroid carcinomas are nonfunctional and may simulate thyroid carcinomas both clinically and pathologically (1,16,18,24).

A high proportion of patients have symptoms attributable to renal disease, with more than two thirds having evidence of nephrolithiasis. In the series reported by Shane and Bilezikian (23), 55 percent of patients had diminished renal function with azotemia and creatinine clearances of less than 50 ml/min (23). In this same series, a similar proportion of patients had evidence of bone disease including osteitis fibrosa cystica, subperiosteal bone resorption, diffuse osteoporosis, "salt and pepper" skull, and absence of the lamina dura.

Patients with parathyroid carcinoma are more likely to present with palpable neck masses than those with adenoma. Up to one third of the patients may have a palpable neck mass at the initial examination (27).

Parathyroid carcinoma is rarely seen in association with familial hyperparathyroidism (14). This association may occur by chance or may represent a generalized tendency in familial disease for progression from hyperplasia to neoplasia.

Gross Features. Parathyroid carcinoma most commonly presents as an ill-defined mass densely adherent to the surrounding soft tissues, thyroid, or periesophageal tissues (fig. 47) (4). Because of this, the surgeon is likely to consider a diagnosis of carcinoma and perform an en bloc resection of the tumor mass at the time of initial surgical exploration. Parathyroid carcinoma, however, can also be encapsulated and can be indistinguishable grossly from adenoma.

In the series reported by Wang and Gaz (27), 13 tumors originated from the upper glands, 11 from the lower glands, and in 4 cases, the exact site of origin could not be determined. The tumors ranged from 1.5 to 6 cm in diameter, with a mean of 3 cm. The mean weight was 6.7 g with a range of 1.5 to 27 g. On section, most tumors were gray-tan, firm,

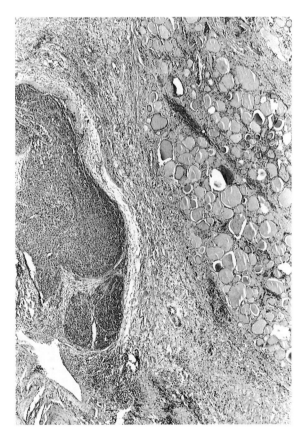

Figure 47
PARATHYROID CARCINOMA
The tumor has invaded the perithyroidal soft tissue.

and ill-defined. Lymph node metastases at the time of initial surgery were uncommon.

In patients with recurrent parathyroid carcinoma, ill-defined masses of firm, gray-tan tissue may be present within and around the previous operative site.

Microscopic Features. The diagnosis of parathyroid carcinoma is often difficult (4,5,15). The histopathologic appearances range from cases that differ minimally from adenoma to those that are obviously anaplastic and invasive malignancies.

As described by Schantz and Castleman (22), the principle features distinguishing parathyroid carcinoma from adenoma are thick fibrous bands, mitotic activity, capsular invasion, and vascular invasion. Although not all these features are necessarily present in any single case, several usually are. Fibrous bands were present in 90 percent of 67 cases studied by these researchers (22). The pattern of fibrous banding in these tumors is, to some extent, reminiscent of that noted in thymomas (fig. 48). Bands of relatively acellular collagenous tissue subdivide the neoplasm into irregularly sized and shaped compartments. Sometimes, the fibrous bands appear to extend directly from the thickened capsule into the substance of the tumor. It should be cautioned, however, that the presence of fibrous bands is not specific for parathyroid carcinoma. Retrogressive changes within an adenoma may result in an appearance that is almost indistinguishable from that seen in a carcinoma. The presence of hemosiderin and chronic inflammatory cells in a parathyroid neoplasm with fibrous banding suggests the possibility of degenerative change within an adenoma (22).

Mitotic activity is present in approximately 80 percent of parathyroid carcinomas (fig. 49). However, mitoses are also evident in parathyroid hyperplasias and adenomas (21,25). Mitoses in excess of 1 per 10 high-power fields may be present in up to 14 percent of otherwise typical adenomas (21,25). In evaluating a parathyroid neoplasm for mitotic activity, pyknotic nuclei should be distinguished from mitotic figures. Only those mitoses which are clearly identifiable should be counted. Mitoses in endothelial cells and other stromal elements should be distinguished clearly from parenchymal mitoses (22).

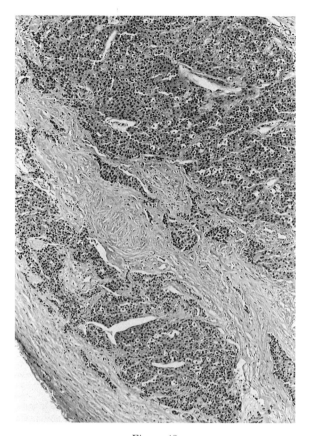

Figure 48
PARATHYROID CARCINOMA
Dense areas of fibrosis extend from the capsule into the substance of the tumor.

The capsules of most carcinomas are thicker than those in adenomas of similar size (fig. 50)(22). Capsular invasion is present in approximately two thirds of parathyroid carcinomas. Invasion can be limited to the capsule or may be evident in the adjacent skeletal muscle, thyroid, or nerve tissue. Invasion in parathyroid neoplasms is characterized by the extension of neoplastic tissue in tongue-like protrusions through the collagenous fibers of the capsule. This should be distinguished from the occasional entrapped clusters of tumor cells which are seen in the capsules of adenomas and are referred to as pseudoinvasion. The latter type of change may be particularly prominent in the capsules of adenomas that have undergone extensive cystic degeneration.

Vascular invasion is seen in approximately 10 to 15 percent of parathyroid carcinomas (figs. 51, 52) (22). This change is particularly evident

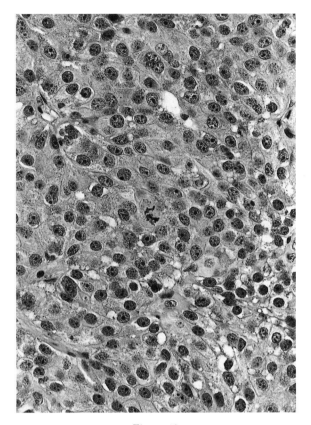

Figure 49
PARATHYROID CARCINOMA
A mitosis is present in the center of the field.

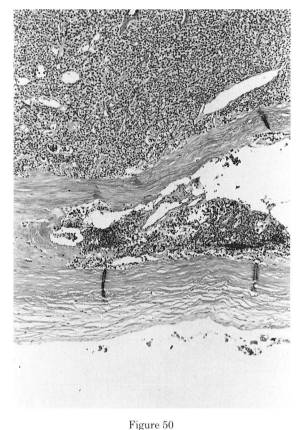

Figure 50
PARATHYROID CARCINOMA
A group of tumor cells has invaded a vascular channel in the capsule of the gland.

within the thickened capsular regions of the tumors. To qualify as bona fide vascular invasion, the tumor must not only be present within a vascular channel but must also be at least partially attached to its wall. Although vascular invasion is not common in parathyroid carcinomas, its presence is virtually diagnostic of malignancy. Invasion of perineural spaces is rarely evident but is a helpful feature when present (fig. 51).

The tumor cells comprising parathyroid carcinomas may be arranged in a trabecular, rosette-like, or sheet-like pattern of growth (figs. 53, 54). Nuclear palisading may be striking in some cases of carcinoma but is also seen in occasional adenomas and hyperplasias. The tumor cells are generally larger than normal chief cells and their nuclei are round to ovoid (figs. 55–58) (11). Most carcinomas show relatively little variation in nuclear size and shape; however, occasional cases show marked nuclear

pleomorphism with coarsely clumped chromatin and prominent nucleoli (figs. 57, 58).

The cytoplasm of parathyroid carcinoma cells may appear relatively clear or eosinophilic and granular (fig. 58, pl. X). The latter appearance suggests oncocytic change in the tumor cells, and these tumors have been referred to as oncocytic variants of parathyroid carcinoma (17).

Although DNA flow cytometric methods have revealed a somewhat greater frequency of aneuploidy in carcinomas, there is considerable overlap with adenomas (13). The studies of Harlow and co-workers (10) suggest that a diagnosis of carcinoma be considered in the presence of an S-phase fraction of greater than 4 percent and a DNA index greater than 1.2

There are relatively few studies of the ultrastructure of parathyroid carcinoma (2,6,17). Some cells have extensively developed Golgi regions with numerous prosecretory granules and

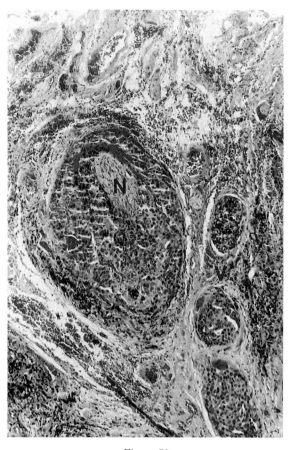

Figure 51
PARATHYROID CARCINOMA
Both vascular (V) invasion and perineural space (N) invasion are present.

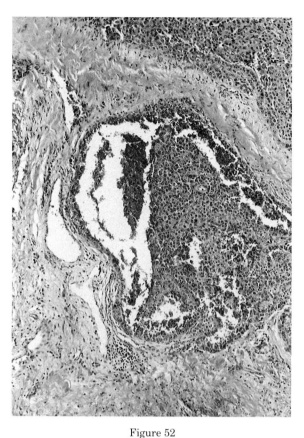

Figure 52
PARATHYROID CARCINOMA
Vascular invasion is present in the soft tissue surrounding the parathyroid.

Figure 53
PARATHYROID
CARCINOMA
The cells are arranged focally in a trabecular pattern.

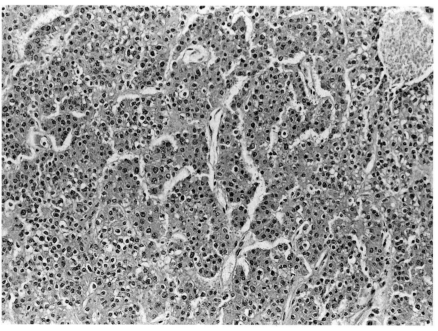

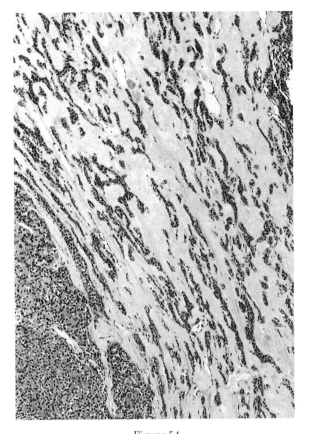

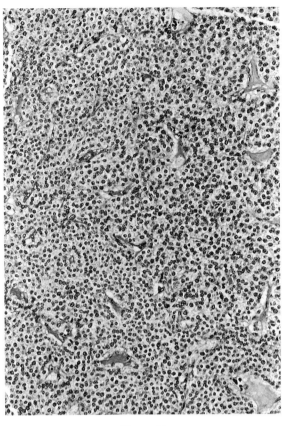

Figure 54
PARATHYROID CARCINOMA
The tumor cells are separated by bands of fibrous connective tissue and are arranged in a trabecular pattern.

Figure 55
PARATHYROID CARCINOMA
This tumor is composed of sheets of uniform chief cells.

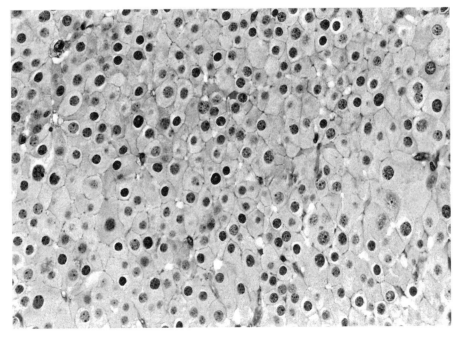

Figure 56
PARATHYROID
CARCINOMA
These tumor cells show moderate variation in nuclear size.

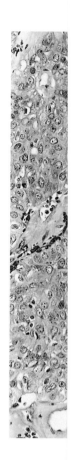

This tum
(Figures 57 :

mature sec
granular e
terna dispe
case from
of the tum
numerous
tracytopla

Differe
of parathy
noma is of
mas are ge
more likel
tissues of t

Charact
mas includ
mitotic act
sular inva
these featu
cific but o

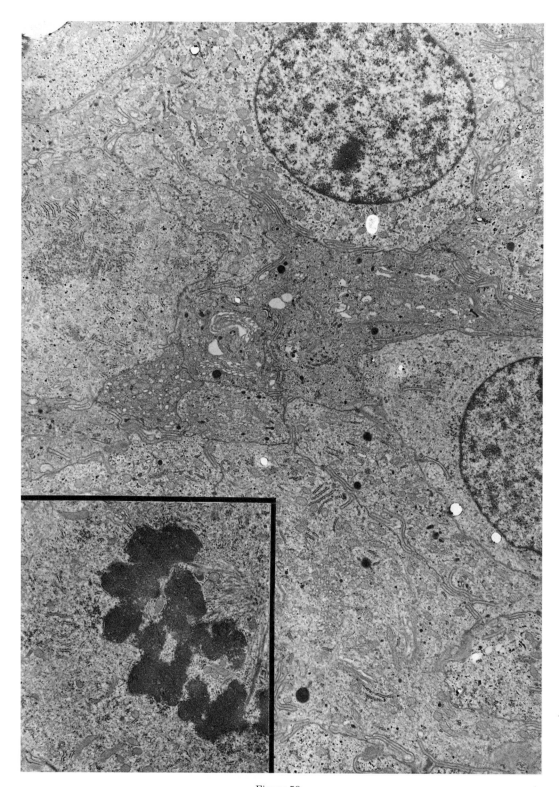

Figure 59
ELECTRON MICROGRAPH OF PARATHYROID CARCINOMA
There are extensive interdigitations of the plasma membranes. There are prominent stacks of granular endoplasmic reticula, and occasional secretory granules are present (X9,000). Inset: mitotic figure (X12,000).

patients had recurrent adenomas containing fragments of suture material at sites of previously excised adenomas.

Microscopic examination of benign implanted parathyroid tissue has failed to show prominent mitotic activity or vascular invasion (20). In patients with true locally recurrent carcinomas, histologic examination shows extensive invasion of surrounding soft tissues and thyroid, vascular invasion, and prominent mitotic activity.

Although the presence of fibrous bands is a feature of parathyroid carcinoma, extensive areas of fibrosis may sometimes be seen in parathyroid adenomas as a retrogressive change. Fibrotic areas within adenomas, in contrast to those in carcinomas, are often accompanied by chronic inflammation and hemosiderin deposition.

The presence of mitoses within a parathyroid adenoma is considered to represent a feature of malignancy. However, the studies of Snover and Foucar (25), and San Juan and co-workers (21), demonstrated mitotic activity in excess of 1 mitosis per 10 high-power fields in up to 14 percent of adenomas. The presence of atypical mitoses, on the other hand, is virtually diagnostic of malignancy.

Clusters of large atypical cells may occur within adenomas. Such cellular clusters appear adjacent to foci of hemorrhage, and their presence should not be used as a criterion in favor of a diagnosis of carcinoma. In fact, such foci are more indicative of adenoma.

There remains a group of parathyroid neoplasms that lacks unequivocal evidence of malignancy, such as vascular or soft tissue invasion (12). These neoplasms are classified by some authors as atypical adenomas, as discussed on pp. 48 and 49.

Nonfunctional parathyroid carcinomas occur and may be misdiagnosed as thyroid carcinomas of either follicular or medullary type. Ordóñez and co-workers (18) reported an intrathyroidal tumor which contained amyloid and mimicked medullary thyroid carcinoma. A positive immunoreaction for parathyroid hormone, negative staining for calcitonin, and a return of the calcium levels to normal after resection confirmed the parathyroid origin of this tumor.

The presence of follicles in nonfunctional parathyroid carcinoma may lead to an erroneous diagnosis of follicular carcinoma of thyroid origin. In a case reported by Ordóñez and co-workers (18), a positive reaction for parathyroid hormone established the diagnosis of parathyroid carcinoma. Oncocytic parathyroid carcinomas may be mistakenly diagnosed as follicular onocytic carcinomas. The latter, however, are typically positive for thyroglobulin and negative for parathyroid hormone.

Treatment. The optimal treatment for patients with parathyroid carcinoma is en bloc resection at the time of initial surgery (8). Failure to remove the adjacent tissues together with the tumor leads to local recurrence in a very high proportion of patients. En bloc resection generally includes removal of the adjacent thyroid lobe, paratracheal soft tissues and lymph nodes, and the ipsilateral thymus (27). A neck dissection is performed only when there is evidence of node involvement. Surgical excision of distant metastases may provide excellent palliation (9).

Prognosis. In the series of 28 patients reported by Wang and Gaz (27), 14 (50 percent) were cured by initial en bloc resection of the tumor. If the tumor recurs, it usually does so within 3 years after the initial surgery. Recurrence is manifested by invasion of contiguous structures including the thyroid, "strap" muscles of the neck, recurrent laryngeal nerve, blood vessels, esophagus, and trachea (fig. 60).

Shane and Bilezikian (23) reported that 35 percent of their patients with parathyroid carinoma ultimately developed metastases. The most common sites of metastases included the cervical lymph nodes (30 percent), lung (40 percent), and liver (10 percent) (fig. 61). Other sites include bone, pleura, and pericardium. In the absence of locally recurrent disease, metastases may be suspected in the presence of persistent hypercalcemia or progressive elevations of parathyroid hormone levels.

Recurrence and metastases are heralded clinically by the development of recurrent hypercalcemia (26). Most parathyroid carcinomas are relatively slow-growing neoplasms. Because of this indolent behavior, surgical excision of metastases may provide excellent palliation. The average survival in patients with recurrence is 7 to 8 years. A variety of nonsurgical approaches are used to control the associated hypercalcemia, including the administration of calcitonin, diphosphonates, and estrogens (26). The tumors are not generally radioresponsive.

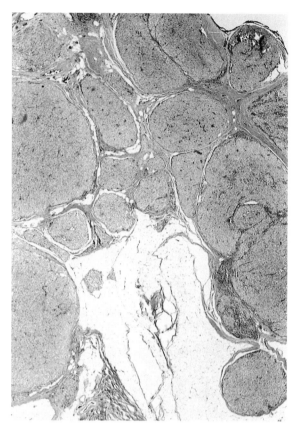

Figure 60
RECURRENT PARATHYROID CARCINOMA
Multiple nodules of recurrent tumor are present in the soft tissue of the neck.

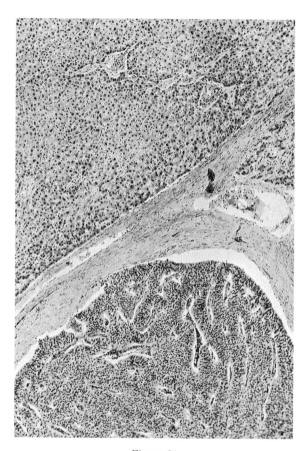

Figure 61
PARATHYROID CARCINOMA
Liver metastasis. (From fig. 38, Fascicle 15, First Series.)

Schantz and Castleman (22) reported that recurrence of tumor within 2 years of diagnosis was a poor prognostic sign. The cause of death was directly or indirectly attributed to parathyroid disease in 72 percent of cases (hyperparathyroidism with severe hypercalcemia, extensive metastases, renal disease, acute pancreatitis).

The value of flow cytometry in distinguishing parathyroid carcinoma from adenoma is controversial (13). However, the studies of Obara and co-workers (15) suggest that flow cytometric analysis of nuclear DNA content is a helpful parameter for the prediction of clinical outcome

in patients with parathyroid carcinoma. In their series, 5 (31 percent) carcinomas were aneuploid. Four of the 5 patients with aneuploid carcinomas had local recurrences or metastases. Four of the 11 patients with diploid carcinomas had either local recurrence or pulmonary metastases, while the remaining 7 patients had no evidence of recurrence 2 to 5 years after initial surgery. These findings suggest that patients with aneuploid parathyroid carcinomas are likely to show a more aggressive form of the disease than those with diploid carcinomas.

REFERENCES

1. Aldinger KA, Hickey RC, Ibanez ML, Samaan NA. Parathyroid carcinoma: a clinical study of seven cases of functioning and two cases of nonfunctioning parathyroid cancer. Cancer 1982;49:388–97.

2. Altenähr E, Saeger W. Light and electron microscopy of parathyroid carcinoma. Report of 3 cases. Virchows Arch [A] 1973;360:107–22.

3. Black BK. Carcinoma of the parathyroid. Ann Surg 1954;139:355-63.

4. Castleman B, Roth SI. Tumors of the parathyroid glands. Atlas of Tumor Pathology, 2nd Series, Fascicle 14. Washington, D.C.: Armed Forces Institute of Pathology, 1978, 1–94.

5. de la Garza S, Flores de la Garza E, Hernández-Batres F. Functional parathyroid carcinoma. Cytology, histology and ultrastructure of a case. Diagn Cytopathol 1985;1:232–5.

6. Faccini JM. The ultrastructure of parathyroid glands removed from patients with primary hyperparathyroidism: a report of 40 cases, including four carcinomata. J Pathol 1970;102:189–99.

7. Fitko R, Roth SI, Hines JR, Roxe DM, Cahill E. Parathyromatosis in hyperparathyroidism. Hum Pathol 1990;21:234–7.

8. Fujimoto Y, Obara T. How to recognize and treat parathyroid carcinoma. Surg Clin North Am 1987;67:343–57.

9. _____, Obara T, Ito Y, Kodama T, Nobori M, Ebihara S. Localization and surgical resection of metastatic parathyroid carcinoma. World J Surg 1986;10:539–47.

10. Harlow S, Roth SI, Bauer K, Marshall RB. Flow cytometric DNA analysis of normal and pathologic parathyroid glands. Mod Pathol 1991;4:310–5.

11. Jacobi JM, Lloyd HM, Smith JF. Nuclear diameter in parathyroid carcinomas. J Clin Pathol 1986;39:1353–4.

12. Levin KE, Galante M, Clark OH. Parathyroid carcinoma versus parathyroid adenoma in patients with profound hypercalcemia. Surgery 1987;101:649–60.

13. Mallette LE. DNA quantitation in the study of parathyroid lesions. A review. Am J Clin Pathol 1992;98:305–11.

14. _____, Bilezikian JP, Ketcham AS, Aurbach GD. Parathyroid carcinoma in familial hyperparathyroidism. Am J Med 1974;57:642–8.

15. McKeown PP, McGarity WC, Sewell CW. Carcinoma of the parathyroid gland: is it over diagnosed? A report of three cases. Am J Surg 1984;147:292–8.

16. Murphy MN, Glennon PG, Diocee MS, Wick MR, Cavers DJ. Nonsecretory parathyroid carcinoma of the mediastinum. Light microscopic, immunocytochemical, and ultrastructural features of a case, and a review of the literature. Cancer 1986;58:2468–76.

17. Obara T, Fujimoto Y, Yamaguchi K, Takanashi R, Kino I, Sasaki Y. Parathyroid carcinoma of the oxyphil cell type. A report of two cases, light and electron microscopic study. Cancer 1985;55:1482–9.

18. Ordóñez NG, Samaan NA, Ibáñez ML, Hickey RC. Immunoperoxidase study of uncommon parathyroid tumors. Report of 2 cases of nonfunctioning parathyroid carcinoma in one intrathyroid parathyroid tumor-producing amyloid. Am J Surg Pathol 1983;7:535–42.

19. Palmer JA, Rosen IB. Reoperative surgery for hyperparathyroidism. Am J Surg 1982;144:406–10.

20. Rattner DW, Marrone GC, Kasdon E, Silen W. Recurrent hyperparathyroidism due to implantation of parathyroid tissue. Am J Surg 1985;149:745–8.

21. San Juan J, Monteagudo C, Fraker D, Norton J, Merino M. Significance of mitotic activity and other morphologic parameters in parathyroid adenomas and their correlation with clinical behavior [Abstract]. Am J Clin Pathol 1989;92:523.

22. Schantz A, Castleman B. Parathyroid carcinoma. A study of 70 cases. Cancer 1973;31:600–5.

23. Shane E, Bilezikian JP. Parathyroid carcinoma: a review of 62 patients. Endocr Rev 1982;3:218–26.

24. Sieracki JC, Horn RC. Nonfunctional carcinoma of the parathyroid. Cancer 1960;13:502–6.

25. Snover DC, Foucar K. Mitotic activity in benign parathyroid disease. Am J Clin Pathol 1981;75:345–7.

26. Trigonis C, Cedermark B, Willems J, Hamberger B, Granberg PO. Parathyroid carcinoma—problems in diagnosis and treatment. Clin Oncol 1984;10:11–9.

27. Wang CA, Gaz RD. Natural history of parathyroid carcinoma. Diagnosis, treatment and results. Am J Surg 1985;149:522–7.

PRIMARY CHIEF CELL HYPERPLASIA

Definition. An absolute increase in parathyroid parenchymal cell mass resulting from proliferation of chief cells, oncocytic cells, and transitional oncocytic cells in multiple parathyroid glands in the absence of a known stimulus for parathyroid hormone hypersecretion. Since the proliferating parathyroid parenchymal cells are often arranged in nodules, primary chief cell hyperplasia is also referred to as *nodular hyperplasia* or *multiple adenomatosis*.

General Features. Chief cell hyperplasia was first reported as a cause of primary hyperparathyroidism by Cope and co-workers in 1958 (19). These authors recognized that it was difficult, if not impossible, to distinguish chief cell hyperplasia from adenoma on the basis of the histologic examination of a single enlarged gland.

Biochemically, primary chief cell hyperplasia is characterized by the excessive and inappropriate synthesis and secretion of parathyroid hormone. In most large case series, primary chief cell hyperplasia has been found in approximately 15 percent of patients with primary hyperparathyroidism (16). The stimulus for chief cell proliferation in this disorder, however, is unknown, although some studies have reported the presence of a circulating factor that is mitogenic for parathyroid cells in culture (13,14). Alternatively, primary chief cell hyperplasia may result from a resetting of the level around which alterations in serum calcium concentrations modify the synthesis and secretion of parathyroid hormone.

The prevalence of parathyroid hyperplasia appears to increase with age. Akerström and co-workers (1), for example, found parathyroid hyperplasia in 7 percent of routinely examined parathyroid glands studied at autopsy. Serum calcium levels were increased in subjects with hyperplastic glands containing large nodules. None of the patients had clinical, biochemical, or histologic evidence of advanced renal disease. Although the relationships of parathyroid hyperplasia and neoplasia are unknown, there are some data to support the view that chief cell hyperplasia represents a precursor of parathyroid adenoma (24,27).

Clinical Features. The clinical features in patients with primary chief cell hyperplasia do not differ significantly from those of parathyroid adenoma. Of particular interest and importance, however, is the association of chief cell hyperplasia with the dominantly inherited multiple endocrine neoplasia (MEN) syndromes (20). Approximately 20 percent of patients with primary chief cell hyperplasia have one of the MEN syndromes (Table 3).

Type I MEN syndrome (Wermer syndrome) is characterized by development of synchronous or metachronous tumors, hyperplasias, or both involving the parathyroids, pancreatic islets, and anterior pituitary. Affected patients may also have an increased incidence of bronchogenic and gastrointestinal carcinoids, adrenal cortical adenomas, and thyroid follicular neoplasms. In most series, the parathyroids are the most commonly affected endocrine glands (6). Parathyroid glands from such patients show evidence of chief cell hyperplasia of the diffuse and nodular types, although examples of adenomas and carcinomas have also been documented (3,28).

Molecular studies using restriction fragment length polymorphism analysis reveal that these apparently hyperplastic glands represent, in fact, monoclonal proliferations (5,21). A single inherited locus on chromosome 11, band q13, is most likely responsible for the development of MEN I. Moreover, the monoclonal development of parathyroid and pancreatic islet cell lesions in affected patients involves similar allelic deletions on chromosome 11. The studies of Friedman (21) have further shown that lesions with chromosomal deletions are larger than those without deletions, suggesting that a monoclonal proliferation may develop after a phase of polyclonal hyperplasia. Some sporadic parathyroid adenomas have allelic losses on chromosome 11 which may also involve the MEN I gene.

The locus for the INT2 oncogene and the MEN I locus are closely linked on chromosome 11, suggesting that INT2 may be important in the development of parathyroid tumors. In this regard, INT2 encodes a protein of the fibroblast growth factor family. Plasma from patients with type I MEN contains a factor that is mitogenic for parathyroid chief cells in vitro and may have some similarities to the basic fibroblast growth

Table 3

MULTIPLE ENDOCRINE NEOPLASIA (MEN) SYNDROMES

Syndrome	Components of Syndrome	Frequency of Parathyroid Involvement
MEN I (Wermer Syndrome)	Parathyroid hyperplasia/adenoma, pituitary adenoma, pancreatic endocrine cell hyperplasia/tumor, gastrointestinal endocrine cell hyperplasia/tumor. (Bronchial and thymic carcinoid, adrenal cortical adenoma, thyroid follicular adenoma.)	Common (90%)
MEN IIA (Sipple Syndrome)	C-cell hyperplasia/medullary thyroid carcinoma, adrenal medullary hyperplasia/pheochromocytoma, parathyroid hyperplasia/adenoma.	Intermediate (30–40%)
MEN IIB	C-cell hyperplasia/medullary thyroid carcinoma, adrenal medullary hyperplasia/pheochromocytoma. Gastrointestinal and ocular-cutaneous ganglioneuromatosis, megacolon. Marfanoid habitus, pes cavus, other skeletal abnormalities.	Rare

factor (21). The studies of Brandi (14) suggest that the action of this factor may be mediated via parathyroid endothelial cells.

Type IIA MEN syndrome is characterized by the development of medullary thyroid carcinoma, pheochromocytoma, and parathyroid hyperplasia (20). Type IIB MEN is characterized by the development of pheochromocytoma, medullary thyroid carcinoma, and ocular, oral, and gastrointestinal ganglioneuromatosis. Parathyroid abnormalities have been noted in up to 30 to 40 percent of type IIA MEN patients with pheochromocytoma and medullary thyroid carcinoma, but are typically absent in the type IIB syndrome. In a study of 12 patients from a large kindred with type IIA MEN (mean age 38 years) who underwent thyroidectomy between 1969 and 1971, increased parathyroid hormone concentrations were found in 6, while 10 had histologic evidence of mild parathyroid hyperplasia (23). In 22 patients screened after 1971, the levels of parathyroid hormone did not differ significantly from those of unaffected family controls. Moreover, none of the patients studied after thyroidectomy developed hyperparathyroidism. These findings indicate that parathyroid abnormalities are significantly less common in patients with type IIA MEN than in individuals with the type I syndrome (23).

The gene for the IIA and IIB MEN syndromes has been linked to the pericentromeric region of chromosome 10 (31,43). In addition to the well-defined types I, IIA, and IIB MEN syndromes, mixed or crossover MEN syndromes, in which a component of one disorder is present in combination with elements of another, have been reported (20). Pheochromocytomas, islet cell tumors, or both have been seen in two or more members of three unrelated families in a manner consistent with an autosomal dominant mode of inheritance (15).

Mixed MEN syndromes associated with parathyroid hyperplasia or adenoma have also been reported. Hansen and co-workers (25) noted the association of neurofibromas, medullary thyroid carcinoma, and parathyroid adenomas together with adrenal cortical adenoma and bronchogenic small cell carcinoma. An association exists between eosinophilic pituitary adenomas and pheochromocytomas with or without accompanying parathyroid hyperplasia (20). Berg and co-workers (7) noted the association of chemodectoma, bronchial carcinoid, pituitary adenoma, chief cell hyperplasia of the parathyroid, and gastroduodenal gastrin cell hyperplasia. Parathyroid chief cell hyperplasia has been found in association with pituitary adenomas, multicentric papillary carcinoma of the thyroid, carotid body paragangliomas, and gastric leiomyomas (26). Of interest is the recent report of the association of gastric carcinoid and parathyroid hyperplasia (36).

Familial hyperparathyroidism associated with chief cell hyperplasia or adenomas may also occur without other associated endocrine abnormalities (3,37).

Gross Findings. Black and Haff (8) recognized three major patterns of gland involvement in patients with chief cell hyperplasia: classic, pseudoadenomatous, and occult. In the typical or classic case, all the glands are enlarged to some extent. In the pseudoadenomatous variant, there is considerable variation in the extent of gland enlargement; some glands are only minimally enlarged, while other glands are markedly enlarged (fig. 62). Black and Haff (8) also recognized a so-called "occult" group in which all of the parathyroids were only minimally enlarged and showed subtle microscopic evidence of hyperplasia. The numbers of classic, pseudoadenomatous, and occult hyperplasia cases were approximately equal in their series (8).

Akerström and co-workers (2) reported that in about two thirds of their patients with chief cell hyperplasia no more than two glands were enlarged. In the series reported from the Massachusetts General Hospital (16), about 50 percent of the patients had glands of approximately equal size. In the remaining cases, one gland was significantly larger than the other three. In the same series, the total weight of the glands was less than 1 g in 54 percent of the patients, while 28 percent had a total gland weight of 1 to 5 g. Only 18 percent of the cases had a gland weight of 5 to 10 g and none had a gland weight in excess of 10 g.

Glands that show minimal enlargement may be difficult to distinguish from normal glands. With increasing size, the glands often assume irregular configurations with pseudopodal projections from their surfaces. On cross section, the glands vary from yellow-brown to red. In most cases, cut surfaces appear homogeneous but distinct nodularity may be apparent and cystic change may be evident grossly (18).

Microscopic Findings. Chief cell hyperplasia is characterized by an increased parenchymal cell mass. The predominant cell in this form of hyperplasia is the chief cell, although variable numbers of oncocytic and transitional oncocytic

cells may be present as well (16). Stromal fat cells are markedly decreased. Because of the regional variations in the distribution of stromal fat cells, however, small biopsies of hyperplastic glands may show a normal chief cell to stromal fat ratio in some foci (16,45).

Although primary chief cell hyperplasia may show either a diffuse or nodular pattern of growth, the nodular variety is more common (figs. 63, 64). Nodular hyperplasia may be particularly evident early in the evolution of the disease. The nodular foci contain few or no stromal fat cells, while the internodular and perinodular regions contain more numerous stromal fat cells (figs. 65, 66). Fibrous septa may surround the nodules in some cases.

Occasionally, cases of primary chief cell hyperplasia have abundant stromal fat cells, and biopsies of such glands can lead to an erroneous diagnosis of a normocellular gland. If the pathologist has not examined the intact glands grossly, it may not be evident that they are enlarged. Strauss and co-workers (45) introduced the term *lipohyperplasia* to describe such hyperplastic glands with abundant stromal fat (fig. 67). Most of the resected glands in their series weighed between 100 and 200 mg, with the largest gland weighing 820 mg.

Multifocal aggregates of hyperplastic chief cells may also be evident in the soft tissues of the neck and mediastinum in patients with primary chief cell hyperplasia (fig. 68). In a study reported by Reddick (35), 3 of 40 patients with primary chief cell hyperplasia had evidence of multiple parathyroid nests in the soft tissues of the neck or mediastinum. These lesions are referred to as *parathyromatosis*, and they may be responsible for persistent or recurrent hyperparathyroidism in patients treated by subtotal parathyroidectomy for chief cell hyperplasia. Parathyromatosis probably results from stimulation of embryonic nests of parathyroid cells in individuals with primary hyperparathyroidism. Supernumerary parathyroid glands also become hyperplastic in patients with primary chief cell hyperplasia (41).

Hyperplastic cells may be arranged in solid sheets, cords, or follicles (figs. 69–72). Proliferating chief cells, which can appear slightly larger than normal chief cells, generally predominate, and increased numbers of oncocytic and transitional oncocytic cells may also be evident. Nodules may

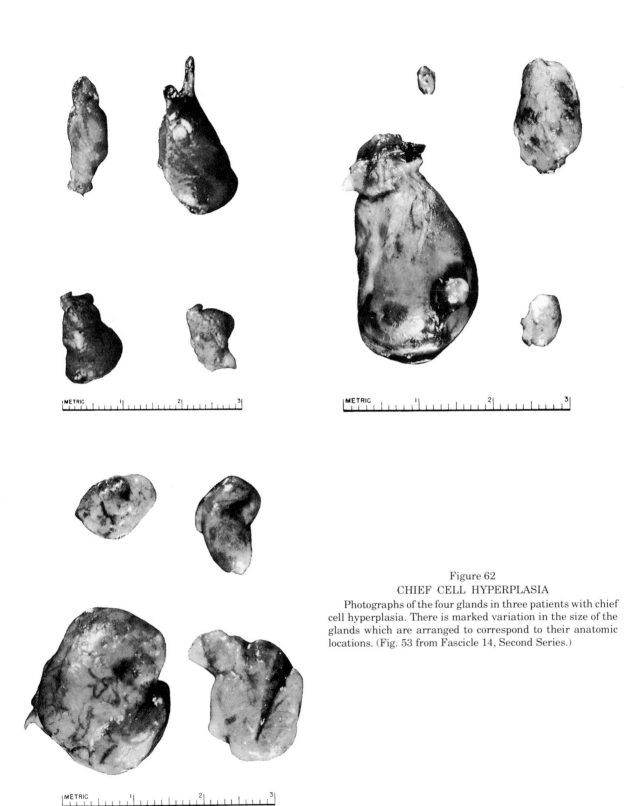

Figure 62
CHIEF CELL HYPERPLASIA
Photographs of the four glands in three patients with chief cell hyperplasia. There is marked variation in the size of the glands which are arranged to correspond to their anatomic locations. (Fig. 53 from Fascicle 14, Second Series.)

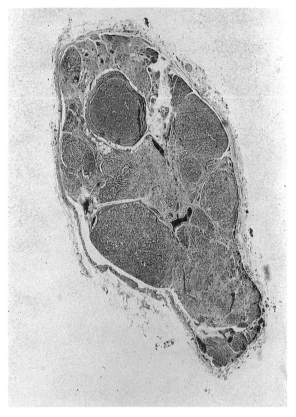

Figure 63
PRIMARY CHIEF CELL HYPERPLASIA
In the nodular type of hyperplasia, associated with type
I MEN, the nodules are present throughout the gland.
(Figures 63 and 64 are from the same patient.)

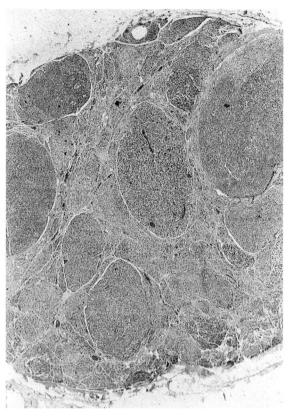

Figure 64
PRIMARY CHIEF CELL HYPERPLASIA
In the nodular type of hyperplasia, associated with type
I MEN, the nodules show considerable variation in size.

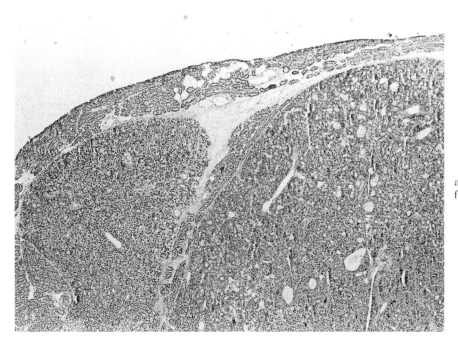

Figure 65
PRIMARY CHIEF CELL
HYPERPLASIA,
NODULAR TYPE
The periphery of the gland
appears compressed with the
formation of a "pseudorim."

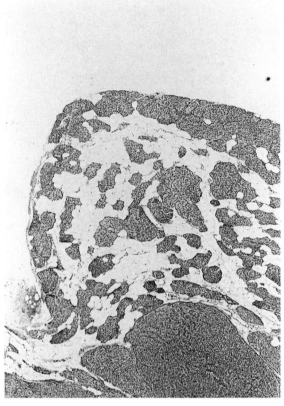

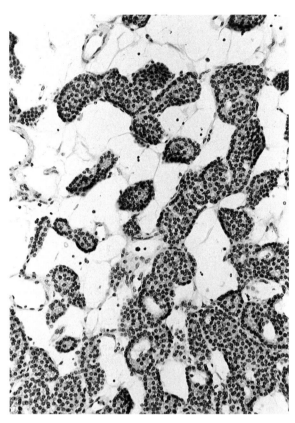

Figure 66
PRIMARY CHIEF CELL HYPERPLASIA
Primary chief cell hyperplasia associated with type I MEN. The parathyroid tissue at the periphery of this hypercellular gland contains abundant stromal fat.

Figure 67
PRIMARY CHIEF CELL HYPERPLASIA
This gland contains abundant stromal fat.

Figure 68
PRIMARY CHIEF CELL
HYPERPLASIA
Clusters of hyperplastic chief cells (parathyromatosis) are present in the soft tissue adjacent to one of the enlarged parathyroid glands.

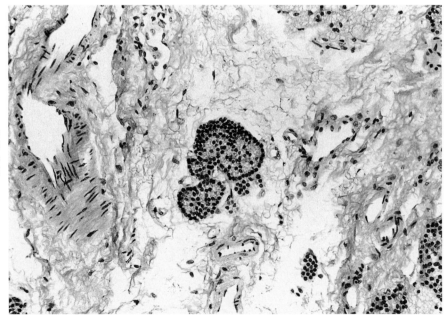

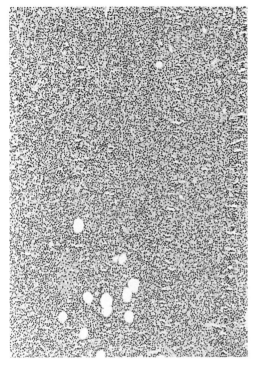

Figure 69
PRIMARY CHIEF CELL HYPERPLASIA
This gland shows a predominantly diffuse pattern of growth.
(Figures 69 and 70 are from the same patient.)

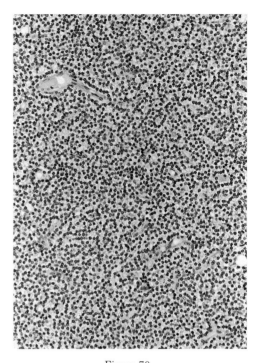

Figure 70
PRIMARY CHIEF CELL HYPERPLASIA
The arrangement of chief cells is identical to that seen
in chief cell adenoma.

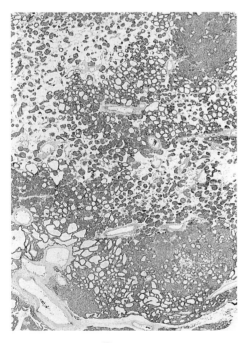

Figure 71
PRIMARY CHIEF CELL HYPERPLASIA
The chief cells are arranged in glandular patterns. (Figures 71 and 72 are from the same patient.)

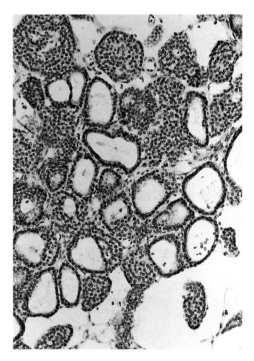

Figure 72
PRIMARY CHIEF CELL HYPERPLASIA
The chief cells are arranged in glandular patterns.

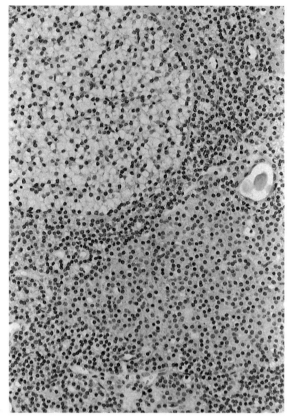

Figure 73
PRIMARY CHIEF CELL HYPERPLASIA
This primary chief cell hyperplasia is predominantly diffuse with two areas of nodularity. The upper nodule is composed of vacuolated chief cells, while the lower nodule is composed of transitional oncocytic cells.

per 10 high-power fields, while 20 percent had more than 1 per 10 high-power fields. The highest degree of mitotic activity (5 mitoses per 10 high-power fields) was found in a case of hyperplasia associated with type IIA MEN. There was no mitotic activity in 20 percent of the cases,

Hyperplastic parathyroid cells may show slight variation in nuclear size and shape with occasional enlarged hyperchromatic nuclei. Pronounced degrees of nuclear pleomorphism, however, are more typical of adenomas. Hyperplastic glands, particularly if they are markedly enlarged, may also show evidence of fibrosis and hemosiderin deposition.

Chronic parathyroiditis is rarely found in association with primary chief cell hyperplasia (10, 12). In two cases reported by Bondeson and associates (10), dense accumulations of lymphocytes were noted within the stroma of hyperplastic parathyroid tissue. In some areas the stroma was densely fibrotic while other areas had a loose and edematous texture. Foci of lymphoid follicle formation, plasmacytic infiltration, and areas of parenchymal destruction were also noted. In contrast to the focal perivascular lymphocytic infiltrates encountered in some normal parathyroid glands at autopsy, the extent of lymphocytic infiltration was more extensive in these cases. Although the origin of the lymphocytic infiltration in cases of human parathyroiditis is unknown, it has been suggested that this disorder may have an autoimmune origin. Chronic parathyroiditis has been reported in rabbits after exposure to ozone.

Cystic changes in primary chief cell hyperplasia are uncommon (18). Foci of cystic change, when present, are most likely to occur in very large hyperplastic glands. Mallette and associates (29) have reported an unusual familial variant of primary cystic chief cell hyperplasia.

Ultrastructural Findings. Ultrastructural analyses reveal that most cases of chief cell hyperplasia contain admixtures of chief cells, oncocytic cells, and transitional oncocytic cells (figs. 74, 75) (4,17,33,39). Generally, hyperplastic chief cells are larger than normal chief cells and have more complex interdigitating plasma membranes. Mitochondria are more numerous, the amount of endoplasmic reticulum and Golgi regions is greater, and vesicles both in the Golgi regions and in the cytoplasm are increased. Small numbers of secretory and prosecretory granules

be composed of relatively pure populations of these different cell types (fig. 73). Parathyroid tissue adjacent to nodules contains admixtures of stromal fat cells and chief cells. It is often impossible to distinguish mild forms of diffuse hyperplasia adjacent to a hyperplastic nodule from a rim of parathyroid tissue adjacent to an adenoma (see fig. 66). Fat stains are useful in making this distinction since hyperplastic chief cells usually contain decreased amounts of parenchymal cell fat as compared to normal or suppressed chief cells (pl. XI). Sometimes, however, hyperplastic glands contain abundant parenchymal cell fat.

Occasionally, mitotic figures are found in cases of chief cell hyperplasia (42,44). Snover and Foucar (42) reported mitoses in 80 percent of cases of primary and secondary hyperplasia; 60 percent of cases had less than 1 mitotic figure

PLATE XI

CHIEF CELL HYPERPLASIA

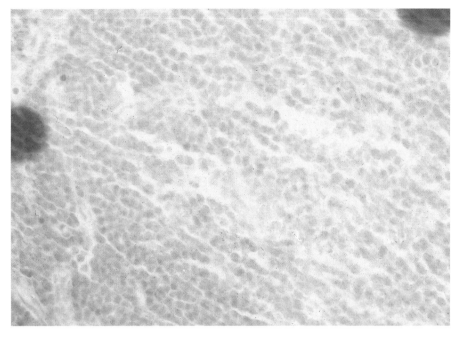

A. This gland contains a very small amount of intraparenchymal fat. Frozen section stained with oil red O.

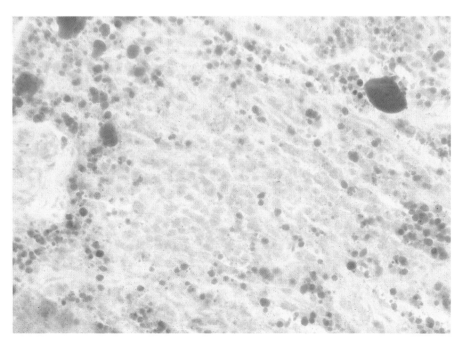

B. This gland contains abundant intraparenchymal fat. A few groups of parenchymal cells are devoid of fat. Frozen section stained with oil red O.

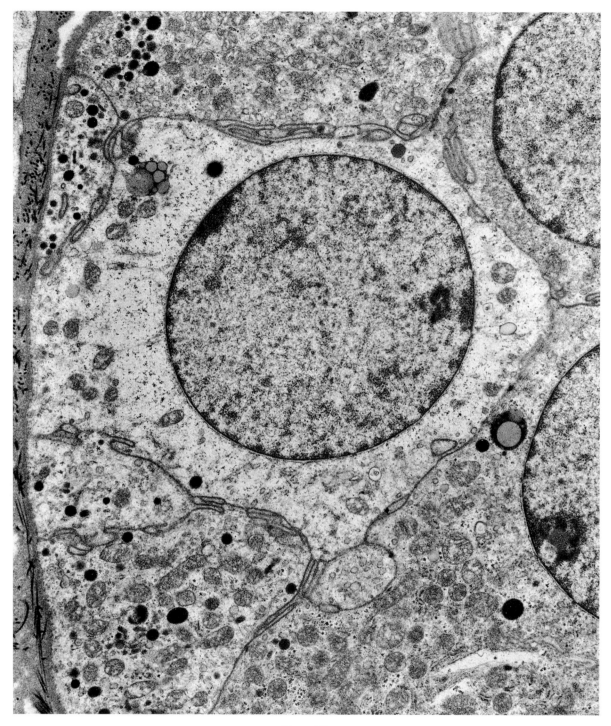

Figure 74
ELECTRON MICROGRAPH OF PRIMARY CHIEF CELL HYPERPLASIA
The plasma membranes show focally complex interdigitations. Moderate numbers of secretory granules are present as well as occasional lipid droplets (X11,400).

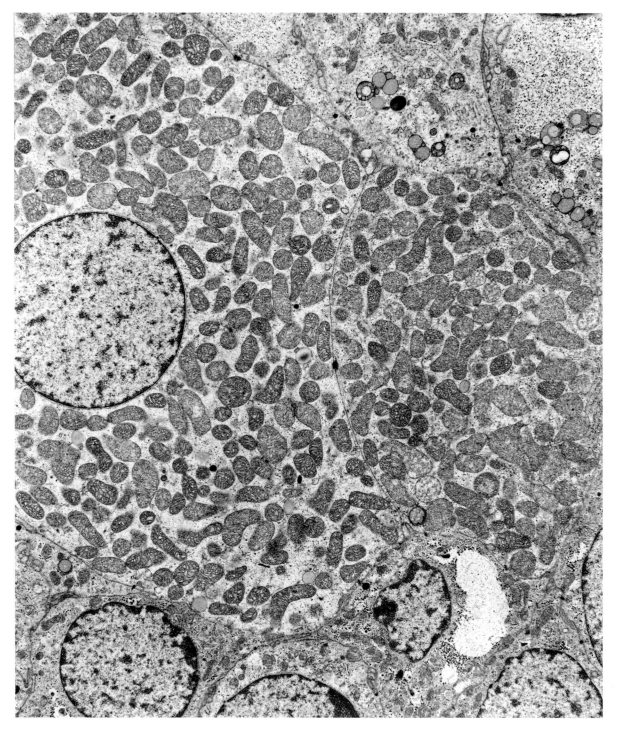

Figure 75
ELECTRON MICROGRAPH OF PRIMARY CHIEF CELL HYPERPLASIA
Occasional small groups of transitional oncocytic cells are present (X6,840).

have been noted. As compared to controls, hyperplastic cells contain more abundant glycogen but smaller amounts of cytoplasmic lipid.

The diagnosis of hyperplasia is particularly difficult in children since their parathyroids contain very little stromal fat. A diagnosis of hyperplasia can be made confidently only if total glandular weights are increased.

Differential Diagnosis. Parathyroid hyperplasia must be distinguished from parathyroid adenoma, and knowledge of the surgical findings is essential for this distinction. In primary chief cell hyperplasia, enlargement of at least two parathyroid glands is usually apparent grossly. In contrast, the vast majority of adenomas involve a single gland. Thus, the presence of a single enlarged gland together with the finding of three normal sized glands is virtually diagnostic of adenoma. Histologic examination of one of the normal sized parathyroid glands should show a normal parenchymal cell to fat cell ratio.

The presence of a rim of normal parathyroid tissue has been considered an important criterion for distinguishing adenoma from hyperplasia. However, it should be remembered that a rim may not be found in all adenomas, particularly those of large size. In the absence of a rim, it is impossible to distinguish an adenoma from diffuse chief cell hyperplasia. Intraoperative fat stains are not useful in this situation since both hyperplastic and neoplastic chief cells typically have reduced amounts of intraparenchymal fat. Occasionally, however, a fat stain may accentuate a rim of parathyroid tissue adjacent to an adenoma that is not apparent by hematoxylin and eosin staining.

In a patient with a single enlarged gland, examination of a second gland is crucial for the appropriate classification of the disease into the adenoma or hyperplasia categories. If the second gland is of normal size and normal cellularity, the enlarged gland most likely represents an adenoma. The demonstration of abundant intraparenchymal fat in a biopsy of a normal sized parathyroid suggests that the gland is suppressed (11,38). Such an observation further supports the diagnosis of adenoma in the enlarged gland. However, it should be recognized that occasional hyperplastic glands may show prominent deposits of intraparenchymal fat (see pl. XI) (11).

Chief cell hyperplasia, particularly the nodular type, may exhibit portions of compressed, mildly hyperplastic parathyroid parenchyma at the periphery, referred to as "pseudorims" (9). Such areas are often impossible to distinguish from a compressed rim of parathyroid tissue adjacent to an adenoma. Although the pseudorims of hyperplastic glands should have a relatively low fat content, abundant intraparenchymal fat may be observed in some cases (11).

The biopsy results of a second gland in a patient with hyperplasia should also show evidence of hyperplasia. However, some hyperplastic glands are normal or only slightly enlarged. Although intraoperative fat stains are expected to show decreased parenchymal fat in hyperplastic glands, this is not always the case since some hyperplastic glands contain prominent intraparenchymal accumulations of fat. Bondeson (11) has shown that hyperplastic parathyroid tissue, in contrast to normal or suppressed glands, is likely to have divergent areas of fat staining. Thus, some areas of hyperplastic parathyroid contain prominent parenchymal fat deposits, while other areas are devoid of fat (pl. XI).

Bondeson and co-workers (11) have further shown that access to two complete glands and the use of fat stains allows highly reproducible and reliable distinction of adenoma and hyperplasia. Equivocal findings were seen in only 8 percent of cases. As with other special procedures, fat stains should not be used alone for the evaluation of parathyroids. The combined use of fat stains and careful morphologic assessment provides an optimal approach to the analysis of parathyroid disease.

Density gradient measurements are also used for the evaluation of the parenchymal cell content of glands with chief cell hyperplasia.

Prognosis and Treatment. The treatment of choice for patients with chief cell hyperplasia is subtotal parathyroidectomy (30,32). Generally, three entire glands and a portion of the fourth gland are excised, leaving a well-vascularized remnant of 50 to 80 mg. Each thymic tongue is also excised in order to ensure that all parathyroid tissue has been removed. In cases of familial hyperparathyroidism, some surgeons advocate total parathyroidectomy with autotransplantation of approximately 50 mg of parathyroid tissue to the forearm (46).

In patients treated by subtotal parathyroidectomy, recurrent hypercalcemia occurred in 16 percent and was noted 1 to 16 years after surgery (40). Inadequate surgery with failure to recognize hyperplasia is the most common cause of recurrent hypercalcemia in patients with primary chief cell hyperplasia. Many of these patients were cured at reoperation by removal of glands that had been left behind during the initial surgical procedure.

A rare cause of recurrent hypercalcemia in patients treated surgically for chief cell hyperplasia is implantation of hyperplastic parathyroid tissue throughout the soft tissues of the neck and less commonly within the mediastinum (34). Parathyromatosis may also be responsible for persistent or recurrent hyperparathyroidism (22).

REFERENCES

1. Akerström G, Rudberg C, Grimelius L, et al. Histologic parathyroid abnormalities in an autopsy series. Hum Pathol 1986;17:520–7.
2. _____, Bergström R, Grimelius L, et al. Relation between changes in clinical and histopathological features of primary hyperparathyroidism. World J Surg 1986;10:696–702.
3. Allo MD, Thompson NW. Familial hyperparathyroidism caused by solitary adenomas. Surgery 1982;92:486–90.
4. Altenähr E, Arps H, Montz R, Dorn G. Quantitative ultrastructural and radioimmunologic assessment of parathyroid gland activity in primary hyperparathyroidism. Lab Invest 1979;41:303–12.
5. Arnold A. Parathyroid adenomas: clonality in benign neoplasia. In: Cossman J, ed. Molecular genetics in cancer diagnosis. New York: Elsevier, 1990:399–408.
6. Benson L, Ljunghall S, Akerström G, Oberg K. Hyperparathyroidism presenting as the first lesion in multiple endocrine neoplasia type 1. Am J Med 1987;82: 731–7.
7. Berg B, Biörklund A, Grimelius L, et al. A new pattern of multiple endocrine adenomatosis: chemodectoma, bronchial carcinoid, G-H producing pituitary adenoma, and hyperplasia of the parathyroid glands, and antral and duodenal gastrin cells. Acta Med Scand 1976; 200:321–6.
8. Black WC, Haff RC. The surgical pathology of parathyroid chief cell hyperplasia. Am J Clin Pathol 1970; 53:565–79.
9. _____, Utley JR. The differential diagnosis of parathyroid adenoma and chief cell hyperplasia. Am J Clin Pathol 1968;49:761–75.
10. Bondeson AG, Bondeson L, Ljungberg O. Chronic parathyroiditis associated with parathyroid hyperplasia and hyperparathyroidism. Am J Surg Pathol 1984;8:211–5.
11. _____, Bondeson L, Ljungberg O, Tibblin S. Fat staining in parathyroid disease—diagnostic value and impact on surgical strategy: clinicopathological analysis of 191 cases. Hum Pathol 1985;16:1255–63.
12. Boyce BF, Doherty VR, Mortimer G. Hyperplastic parathyroiditis—a new autoimmune disease? J Clin Pathol 1982;35:812–4.
13. Brandi ML, Aurbach GD, Fitzpatrick LA, et al. Parathyroid mitogenic activity in plasma from patients with familial multiple endocrine neoplasia type 1. N Engl J Med 1986;314:1287–93.
14. _____. Multiple endocrine neoplasia type I: General features and new insights into etiology. J Endocrinol Invest 1991;14:61–72.
15. Carney JA, Go VL, Gordon H, Northcutt RC, Pearse AG, Sheps SG. Familial pheochromocytoma and islet cell tumor of the pancreas. Am J Med 1980;68:515–21.
16. Castleman B, Roth SI. Tumors of the parathyroid glands. Atlas of Tumor Pathology, 2nd Series, Fascicle 14. Washington, D.C.: Armed Forces Institute of Pathology, 1978, 1–94.
17. Cinti S, Colussi G, Minola E, Dickersin GR. Parathyroid glands in primary hyperparathyroidism: an ultrastructural study of 50 cases. Hum Pathol 1986;17:1036–46.
18. Clark OH. Hyperparathyroidism due to primary cystic parathyroid hyperplasia. Arch Surg 1978;113:748–50.
19. Cope O, Keynes WM, Roth SI, Castleman B. Primary chief-cell hyperplasia of the parathyroid glands: a new entity in the surgery of hyperparathyroidism. Ann Surg 1958;148:375–88.
20. DeLellis RA, Dayal Y, Tischler AS, Lee AK, Wolfe HJ. Multiple endocrine neoplasia (MEN) syndromes: cellular origins and interrelationships. Int Rev Exp Pathol 1986;28:163–215.
21. Friedman E, Sakaguchi K, Bale AE, et al. Clonality of parathyroid tumors in familial multiple endocrine neoplasia type I. N Engl J Med 1989;321:213–18.
22. Fitko R, Roth SI, Hines JR, et al. Parathyromatosis in hyperparathyroidism. Hum Pathol 1990;21:234–7.
23. Gagel RF, Tashjian AH Jr, Cummings T, et al. The clinical outcome of prospective screening for multiple endocrine neoplasia type 2a. N Engl J Med 1988;318:478–84.
24. Golden A, Canary JJ, Kerwin DM. Concurrence of hyperplasia and neoplasia of the parathyroid glands. Am J Med 1965;38:562–78.
25. Hansen OP, Hansen M, Hansen HH, Rose B. Multiple endocrine adenomatosis of mixed type. Acta Med Scand 1976;200:327–31.
26. Larraza-Hernandez O, Albores-Saavedra J, Benavides G, Krause LB, Perez-Merizaldi JC, Ginzo A. Multiple endocrine neoplasia, pituitary adenoma, multicentric papillary thyroid carcinoma, bilateral carotid body paraganglioma, parathyroid hyperplasia, gastric leiomyoma and systemic amyloidosis. Am J Clin Pathol 1982;78:527–32.
27. Kramer WM. Association of parathyroid hyperplasia with neoplasia. Am J Clin Pathol 1970;53:275–83.

28. Mallette LE, Bilezikian JP, Ketcham AS, Aurbach GD. Parathyroid carcinoma in familial hyperparathyroidism. Am J Med 1974;57:642–8.

29. _____, Malini S, Rappaport MP, Kirkland JL. Familial cystic parathyroid adenomatosis. Ann Intern Med 1987;107:54–60.

30. Malmaeus J, Benson L, Johansson H, et al. Parathyroid surgery in the multiple endocrine neoplasia type 1 syndrome: choice of surgical procedure. World J Surg 1986;10:668–72.

31. Mathew CG, Chin KS, Easton DF, et al. A linked genetic marker for multiple endocrine neoplasia type 2A on chromosome 10. Nature 1987;328:527–8.

32. Palmer JA, Brown WA, Kerr WH, Rosen IB, Watters NA. The surgical aspects of hyperparathyroidism. Arch Surg 1975;110:1004–7.

33. Nilsson O. Studies on the ultrastructure of the human parathyroid glands in various pathological conditions. Acta Pathol Microbiol Immunol Scand [A] 1977;263 (Suppl):1–88.

34. Rattner DW, Marrone GC, Kasdon E, Silen W. Recurrent hyperparathyroidism due to implantation of parathyroid tissue. Am J Surg 1985;149:745–8.

35. Reddick RL, Costa JC, Marx SJ. Parathyroid hyperplasia and parathyromatosis [Letter]. Lancet 1977;1:549.

36. Rode J, Dhillon AP, Cotton PB, Wolfe A, O'Riordan JL. Carcinoid of the stomach and primary hyperparathyroidism—a new association. J Clin Pathol 1987;40:546–51.

37. Roth SI. The parathyroid gland. In: Silverberg SG, ed. Principles and practice of surgical pathology, Vol 2. 2nd ed. New York: Churchill Livingstone, 1990:1923–55.

38. _____, Gallagher MJ. The rapid identification of "normal" parathyroid glands by the presence of intracellular fat. Am J Pathol 1976;84:521–8.

39. _____, Munger BL. The cytology of adenomatous, atrophic and hyperplastic parathyroid glands of man. A light and electron-microscopic study. Virchows Arch [A] 1962;335:389–410.

40. Rudberg C, Akerström G, Palmér M, et al. Late results of operation for primary hyperparathyroidism in 441 patients. Surgery 1986;99:643–51.

41. Russell CF, Grant CS, Van Heerden JA. Hyperfunctioning supernumerary parathyroid glands. An occasional cause of hyperparathyroidism. Mayo Clin Proc 1982;57: 121–4.

42. San Juan J, Monteagudo C, Fraker D, Norton J, Merino M. Significance of mitotic activity and other morphologic parameters in parathyroid adenomas and their correlation with clinical behavior [Abstract]. Am J Clin Pathol 1989;92:523.

43. Simpson NE, Kidd KK, Goodfellow PJ, et al. Assignment of multiple endocrine neoplasia type 2A to chromosome 10 by linkage. Nature 1987;328:528–30.

44. Snover DC, Foucar K. Mitotic activity in benign parathyroid disease. Am J Clin Pathol 1981;75:345–7.

45. Straus FH, Kaplan EL, Nishiyama RH, Bigos ST. Five cases of parathyroid lipohyperplasia. Surgery 1983;94: 901–5.

46. Wells SA, Ellis GJ, Gunnells C, et al. Parathyroid autotransplantation in primary parathyroid hyperplasia. N Engl J Med 1976;295:57.

✧✧✧

CLEAR CELL HYPERPLASIA

Definition. A disorder characterized by an absolute increase in parathyroid parenchymal mass resulting from proliferation of vacuolated water-clear (wasserhelle) cells in multiple parathyroid glands, in the absence of a known stimulus for parathyroid hormone hypersecretion.

General and Clinical Features. Clear cell hyperplasia is a rare disorder. Between 1930 and 1975, only 19 patients with this diagnosis were treated at the Massachusetts General Hospital (1,2). Since that time, very few patients with clear cell hyperplasia have been reported (4). Similar to cases of primary hyperparathyroidism diagnosed before 1975, most individuals with clear cell hyperplasia have had evidence of renal calculi or bone disease.

There is no apparent familial incidence of clear cell hyperplasia, and there is no known association with any of the multiple endocrine neoplasia syndromes (6).

Gross Findings. In most patients with clear cell hyperplasia, all parathyroids are enlarged (pl. XII). Occasionally, only three glands are enlarged, and there may be considerable variation in the size of individual glands in any single case. In the series from the Massachusetts General Hospital, almost half of the cases had total gland weights ranging from 10 to 60 g (1,2). The remaining cases had total glandular weights of less than 10 g.

Gland shape tends to be irregular with pseudopodal extensions into the surrounding adipose tissue of the neck (pl. XII). The upper glands tend to be larger than the lower ones. The glands vary from red-brown to brown, and the more severe cases may show foci of cystic change, hemorrhage, and fibrosis.

Microscopic Findings. The cells characteristically show a diffuse pattern of growth. Individual cells are generally polyhedral with distinct plasma membranes. They have an average diameter of 15 to 20 μm but may range from 10 to 40 μm (figs. 76, 77).The nuclei have an average diameter of 8 μm, are frequently multiple, and tend to be round to slightly ovoid and moderately hyperchromatic with an eccentrically placed nucleolus. They also tend to be located at the pole of the cell which is adjacent to the stroma and vessels. This produces a characteristic pattern which has been likened to bunches of berries (2). Isolated nuclei may be markedly enlarged and hyperchromatic.

The cells may be arranged in glandular or tubular configurations (fig. 78). Occasionally, they are composed of cystic structures lined by clear cells, and the centers of such cysts often contain proteinaceous material with degenerated cells.

The cytoplasm has a strikingly clear appearance at low to medium magnifications. The cells, however, are filled with small vacuoles which measure up to 0.8 μm in diameter (fig. 79, pl. XIII). The cells contain moderate amounts of glycogen, but the vacuoles fail to stain for neutral lipids.

Ultrastructural studies confirm that the clear appearance results from the presence of multiple vacuoles which are probably derived from the Golgi vesicles (figs. 79, 80) (5). Some vacuoles contain a dense central material which most likely represents stored parathyroid hormone. The water-clear cells generally contain very little endoplasmic reticulum and there are small numbers of secretory and prosecretory granules.

Dawkins and associates (3) have demonstrated that in cases of clear cell hyperplasia, the concentration of parathyroid hormone, per mg of fresh tissue, is approximately one thousand times lower than in normal glands or chief cell adenomas.

Treatment. The treatment of choice for patients with clear cell hyperplasia is subtotal parathyroidectomy.

PLATE XII

PRIMARY CLEAR CELL HYPERPLASIA

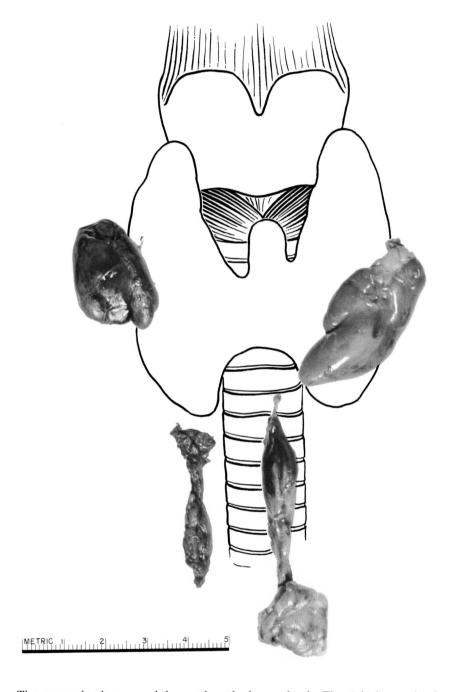

The upper glands are much larger than the lower glands. The right lower gland
is embedded in thymic tissue. (Pl. III from Fascicle 15, First Series.)

PLATE XIII

PRIMARY CLEAR CELL HYPERPLASIA

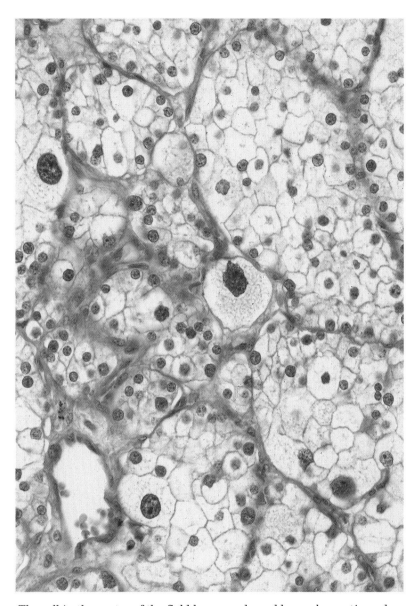

The cell in the center of the field has an enlarged hyperchromatic nucleus and multiple cytoplasmic vacuoles.

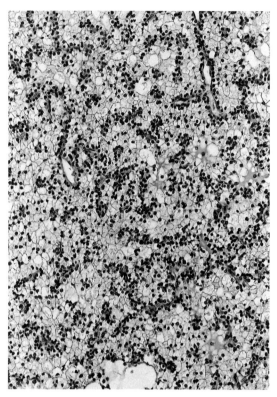

Figure 76
PRIMARY CLEAR CELL HYPERPLASIA
The nuclei are aligned along vascular channels.

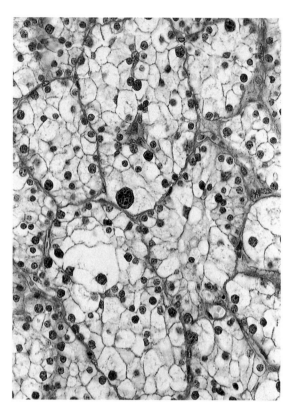

Figure 77
CLEAR CELL HYPERPLASIA
Occasional enlarged, hyperchromatic nuclei are evident.

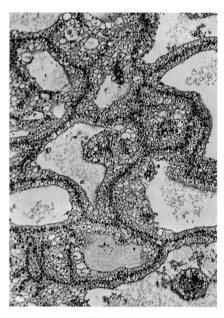

Figure 78
CLEAR CELL HYPERPLASIA
Large cystic spaces containing cellular debris are present. (Fig. 74 from Fascicle 15, First Series.)

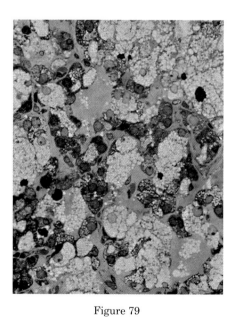

Figure 79
CLEAR CELL HYPERPLASIA
Clear cells contain cytoplasmic vacuoles. Osmium-fixed and epoxy-embedded, 1 μm section stained with toluidine blue. (Fig. 75 from Fascicle 14, Second Series.)

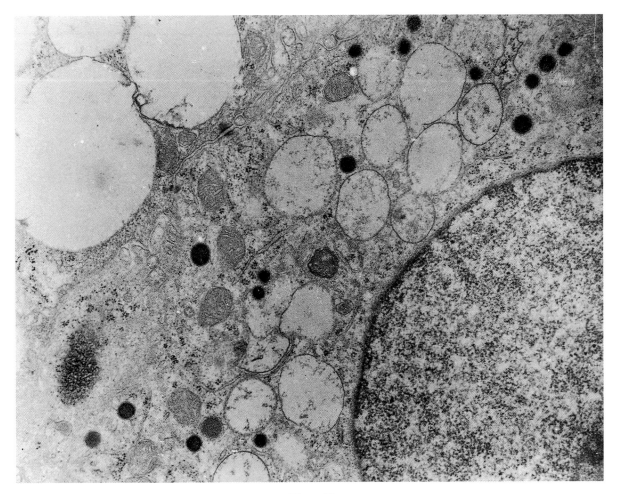

Figure 80
ELECTRON MICROGRAPH OF CLEAR CELL HYPERPLASIA
The cell contains characteristic membrane-limited vacuoles and scattered secretory granules (X22,720). (Fig. 76 from Fascicle 15, First Series.)

REFERENCES

1. Albright F, Bloomberg E, Castleman B, Churchill ED. Hyperparathyroidism due to diffuse hyperplasia of all parathyroid glands rather than adenoma of one. Clinical studies on three such cases. Arch Intern Med 1934;54: 315–29.
2. Castleman R, Roth SI. Tumors of the parathyroid glands. Atlas of Tumor Pathology, 2nd Series, Fascicle 14. Washington, D.C.: Armed Forces Institute of Pathology, 1978, 1–94.
3. Dawkins RL, Tashjian AH Jr, Castleman B, Moore EW. Hyperparathyroidism due to clear cell hyperplasia. Serial determinations of serum ionized calcium, parathyroid hormone and calcitonin. Am J Med 1973;54:119–26.
4. Dorado AE, Hensley G, Castleman B. Water clear cell hyperplasia of parathyroid: autopsy report of a case with supernumerary glands. Cancer 1976;38:1676–83.
5. Roth SI. The ultrastructure of primary water-clear cell hyperplasia of the parathyroid glands. Am J Pathol 1970;61:233–40.
6. Tisell LE, Hedman I, Hansson G. Clinical characteristics and surgical results in hyperparathyroidism caused by water-clear cell hyperplasia. World J Surg 1981; 1981;5:565–71.

SECONDARY AND TERTIARY HYPERPARATHYROIDISM

SECONDARY HYPERPARATHYROIDISM

Definition. An adaptive increase in parathyroid parenchymal mass resulting from a proliferation of chief cells, oncocytic cells, and transitional oncocytic cells in multiple parathyroid glands in the presence of a known stimulus for parathyroid hormone hypersecretion.

Clinical Features. The relationship between chronic renal failure and enlargement of multiple parathyroid glands has been known for many years. In 1935, Pappenheimer and Wilens (12) reported that the parathyroids from patients with chronic renal disease were 50 to 100 percent larger than glands from normal individuals, and these findings were confirmed by other investigators. Increased secretion of parathyroid hormone in this setting results from chronic persistent stimulation of the parathyroids by low levels of ionized calcium in the blood.

Secondary chief cell hyperplasia may also occur in patients with dietary deficiency of vitamin D, abnormal vitamin D metabolism, or pseudohypoparathyroidism. Once the process of parathyroid hyperplasia begins, the set point for the control of parathyroid hormone secretion by ionic calcium rises, and this leads to further hyperplasia and hypersecretion of the hormone (4,14).

The clinical manifestations in patients with secondary hyperparathyroidism are dominated by the presence of skeletal pain and deformities arising from the increased secretion of parathyroid hormone and the diminished synthesis of $1,25(OH)_2D_3$ (14). Osteitis fibrosa cystica and osteomalacia are evident on examination of the bones. Bone disease characterized by normal osteoid volume, absence of fibrosis, and a reduced rate of bone formation has also been described. This disorder may result from accumulation of high levels of aluminum in bone, presumably due to the aluminum contained in dialysis fluids.

Extensive visceral, soft tissue, and periarticular calcifications also occur in patients with chronic renal failure (14). Thus, pain, swelling, and joint stiffness may result in severe disabling arthritis because of calcium deposition around the joints. In addition, deposition of calcium in the media of arteries may be evident. Calciphylaxis is a rare syndrome that can develop in patients with chronic renal failure. It is characterized by ischemic necrosis of the skin, muscles, and subcutaneous fat.

Gross Findings. The appearance of the parathyroid glands in patients with secondary hyperparathyroidism is generally similar to that seen in patients with primary chief cell hyperplasia (pl. XIV-A) (1,6,13). There is a greater tendency, however, for the parathyroid glands in patients with secondary hyperplasia to be more uniform in size early in the course of the disease, than in patients with primary chief cell hyperplasia. In advanced secondary hyperplasia, variation in gland size may be marked. The extent of the hyperplasia generally parallels the severity of the underlying condition which predisposes the patient to secondary hyperparathyroidism, most commonly chronic renal failure.

Generally, the glands in patients with mild secondary hyperparathyroidism are uniformly enlarged and are yellow-tan to creamy gray in color. In 200 cases reported by Roth and Marshall (13), gland weights varied from 120 to 6,000 mg. The glands were firmer and less pliable than normal glands or adenomas.

Microscopic Findings. The earliest change in the parathyroids is a decrease in the number of stromal fat cells and their partial replacement by widened cords and nests of chief cells (figs. 81–83) (13). Most commonly, the proliferating chief cells are present in diffuse sheets, but other areas may show cord-like, acinar, or trabecular patterns of growth (fig. 84).

Advanced stages of secondary hyperplasia are characterized by nodular proliferation of chief cells and oncocytes (figs. 85, 86). The foci of nodular proliferation may be surrounded by a fibrous tissue capsule. Foci of fibrosis, hemorrhage, chronic inflammation, and cyst formation may be evident.

PLATE XIV

SECONDARY AND TERTIARY HYPERPARATHYROIDISM

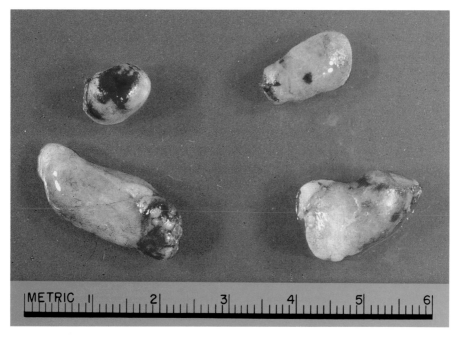

A. Hyperplastic parathyroid glands from a patient with chronic renal failure and secondary hyperparathyroidism. All glands are enlarged.

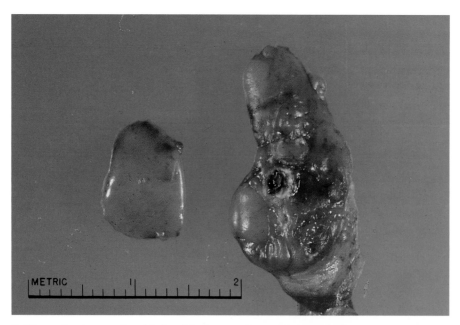

B. Hyperplastic parathyroid gland from a patient with tertiary hyperparathyroidism. This bisected gland shows nodular hyperplasia with foci of calcification and hemorrhage.

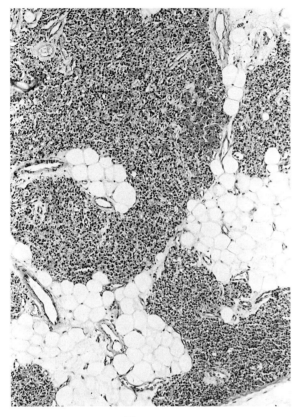

Figure 81
SECONDARY HYPERPARATHYROIDISM
The cords of chief cells are markedly widened.

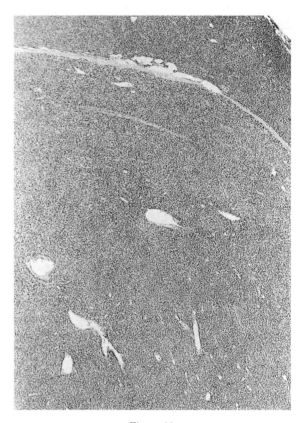

Figure 82
SECONDARY HYPERPARATHYROIDISM
This gland shows a predominantly diffuse pattern of chief cell hyperplasia.

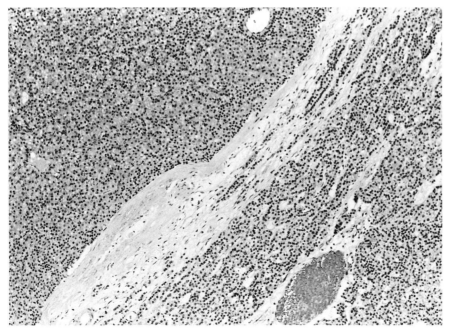

Figure 83
SECONDARY
HYPERPARATHYROIDISM
Areas of fibrosis are noted within the gland.

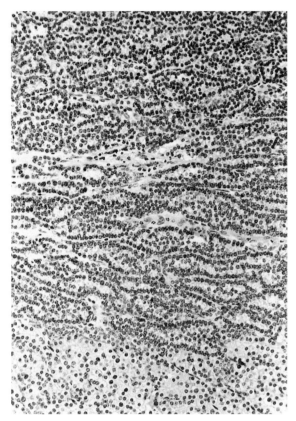

Figure 84
SECONDARY HYPERPARATHYROIDISM
The chief cells show a trabecular pattern of growth.

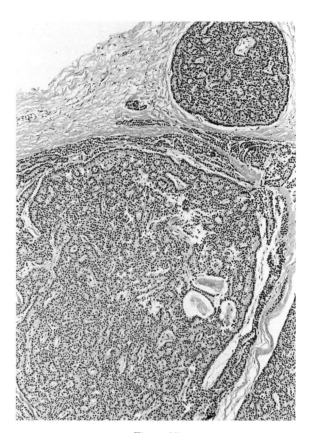

Figure 85
SECONDARY HYPERPARATHYROIDISM
The chief cells show a focal "adenomatoid" pattern of growth.

Figure 86
SECONDARY
HYPERPARATHYROIDISM
Many nodules in this gland
are composed of oncocytic cells.

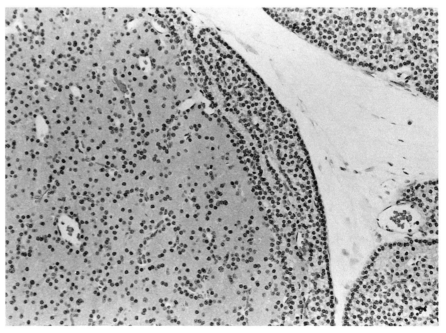

The characteristic cell in secondary hyperplasia is the vacuolated chief cell which measures 6 to 8 µm in diameter (13). The nucleus is small, dense, and occupies a somewhat eccentric position within the cytoplasm (3). Vacuolated chief cells are typically rich in glycogen, and cytoplasmic fat content is reduced.

In addition to chief cells, the parathyroids also contain increased numbers of oncocytic cells and transitional oncocytic cells (fig. 86). In some cases, the chief cells assume a distinctive organoid or adenomatoid pattern of growth (fig. 85) (13).

Harlow and co-workers (8) have reported the presence of aneuploid populations in 4 of 18 glands (22 percent) resected from 5 patients with secondary hyperparathyroidism.

Ultrastructural Findings. Ultrastructural studies have revealed that chief cells have relatively straight plasma membranes with occasional desmosomal attachment sites (9). Roth and Marshall (13) noted that the cytoplasm is relatively electron transparent with occasional parallel cisternae of granular endoplasmic reticula. Numerous secretory granules may be present adjacent to the Golgi regions or plasma membranes.

Oncocytes and transitional oncocytic cells appear to be increased in proportion to the extent of functional renal impairment. Parenchymal fat content is markedly reduced or absent.

Prognosis and Treatment. Surgery for secondary hyperparathyroidism includes subtotal parathyroidectomy with approximately 50 mg of parathyroid tissue left in situ (4). Since the stimulus for parathyroid hyperplasia (chronic renal failure) is still present, the residuum of parathyroid tissue in the neck may eventually become hyperplastic and the patient may require surgical re-exploration. Residual parathyroid tissue may show considerable mitotic activity.

Inadvertent implantation of parathyroid tissue in the soft tissues of the neck at the initial surgery may also be responsible for the recurrence of hyperparathyroidism in the postoperative period (7). In some instances, implants of parathyroid tissue are contiguous with previous suture sites.

Patients with secondary hyperparathyroidism have also been treated by total parathyroidectomy with implantation of approximately 50 mg of parathyroid tissue into the muscle of the forearm (19–21).

Parathyroid Grafts in Patients with Secondary Hyperparathyroidism

Total parathyroidectomy with auto transplantation of parathyroid tissue into the muscles of the forearm is a useful technique for the treatment of secondary hyperparathyroidism (20,21). Both graft failure and insufficient graft function resulting in hypoparathyroidism may occur. Occasionally, patients develop recurrent hyperparathyroidism, with serum parathyroid hormone levels highest in the venous blood of the forearm bearing the graft.

Klempa and co-workers (10) noted recurrent hyperparathyroidism in 6 of 42 patients who had forearm autotransplants. Although only 20 to 40 mg of parathyroid tissue had been transplanted, the removed grafts weighed 0.9 to 3.1 g. Compared to the originally excised parathyroid tissue, the nuclei of the transplanted cells were often larger and more irregular. The hyperfunctioning autografts showed a distinct nodular hyperplasia with focal nuclear pleomorphism and clear cytoplasm. In two cases, mitotic activity was apparent. A striking finding was the presence of small nests of parathyroid tissue next to and at some distance from the autograft, within skeletal muscle and connective tissue. These observations indicate that the proliferation of autografted parathyroid tissue may be extreme enough to simulate malignant transformation (10).

TERTIARY HYPERPARATHYROIDISM

Tertiary hyperparathyroidism refers to the development of autonomous parathyroid hyperfunction occurring in patients with previously documented secondary hyperparathyroidism (18).

Hypercalcemia secondary to hyperparathyroidism develops in about one third of kidney transplant recipients as subacute hypercalcemia appearing shortly after transplantation, transient hypercalcemia, or persistent hypercalcemia (16). Subacute hypercalcemia is rare and occurs within the first 3 weeks following transplantation. Since it may result in deteriorating graft function, early parathyroidectomy is required. Transient hypercalcemia is the most common form of hyperparathyroidism after transplantation, but in most cases it resolves spontaneously. Persistent hypercalcemia has been observed in 15 to 50 percent of patients with long-term graft survival.

The mechanisms for the development of tertiary hyperparathyroidism are unknown, although several studies have suggested that it may result from a calcium set point error. According to this hypothesis, the cellular response function is shifted away from normal towards higher calcium concentrations (14). Parathyroid chief cells, which have higher set points of suppression, increase their biosynthetic and secretory activities and are stimulated to divide even at normal calcium concentrations. This chain of events leads to an increased parenchymal parathyroid mass.

There is considerable controversy concerning the underlying changes in parathyroid glands in patients with tertiary hyperparathyroidism. While some authors suggest that hyperplasia is the most common underlying pathology, others believe that adenomas account for the development of tertiary hyperparathyroidism. Haselton and Ali (9) reported that 6 of 10 patients with chronic renal failure had evidence of multiple adenomas developing on a background of hyperplasia.

Krause and Hedinger (11) reviewed the pathologic findings in 128 resected parathyroids from 41 patients with tertiary hyperparathyroidism. Only 5 percent of the patients had adenomas; the others had evidence of hyperplasia. The hyperplasia was predominantly diffuse in 44 percent; the remaining patients had nodular hyperplasia. The average single parathyroid weight for the diffuse group was 0.7 ± 0.4 g, while the glands from patients with nodular hyperplasia had an average weight of 1.4 ± 0.7 g. Gland enlargement in diffuse hyperplasia was symmetric, while the resected glands with nodular hyperplasia often showed an asymmetric appearance (pl. XIV-B).

In this study, histologic examination of glands with diffuse hyperplasia showed proliferation of parenchymal cells throughout the gland with an average stromal fat content of 5 percent. The predominant cell type was the chief cell although oncocytes and transitional oncocytic cells were also evident. Areas of fibrosis, calcification and iron deposition were present in some cases. Nuclear pleomorphism and mitotic activity were rare.

In patients with nodular hyperplasia, individual nodules were composed of chief cells although nodules of oncocytic cells were also seen. Water-clear cells were rare. Overall mitotic activity was low and nuclear pleomorphism slight, except in oncocytic areas. Foci of fibrosis, iron deposition, and calcification were common (figs. 87–89). The parenchymal cells between the nodules revealed evidence of diffuse hyperplasia. Compression of the internodular areas sometimes resulted in the appearance of small atrophic cells in a rim of tissue similar to that of patients with adenoma.

The ultrastructural features of glands with tertiary hyperparathyroidism have been described in detail (2,13). The proliferating chief cells are joined by multiple interdigitations and desmosomes. The cytoplasm is typically rich in granular endoplasmic reticulum with variable numbers of secretory granules having an average diameter of 0.17 µm. Occasionally, Golgi regions are extremely prominent, and there are moderate quantities of partially dissolved glycogen. Both centrioles and cilia are frequent. These observations indicate that the majority of the cells show high secretory activity.

Adenomas rarely occur in patients with tertiary hyperparathyroidism. In the two cases reported by Krause and Hedinger (11), only one gland was markedly enlarged while biopsies of the remaining glands revealed an essentially normocellular pattern. These features are identical to those described in patients without pre-existing secondary hyperparathyroidism (fig. 90).

Krause and Hedinger (11) compared the morphologic features of glands from patients with secondary and tertiary hyperparathyroidism. In general, gland weights were less in patients with secondary hyperparathyroidism (average weight 0.25 g for diffuse hyperplasia and 1.4 g for nodular hyperplasia). In patients with secondary hyperparathyroidism, the parenchymal proliferation was mostly diffuse and dominated by vacuolated chief cells. The chief cells in tertiary hyperparathyroidism were cytologically more diverse, and oncocytic cells were more prominent. Gland nodularity was more common in tertiary hyperparathyroidism.

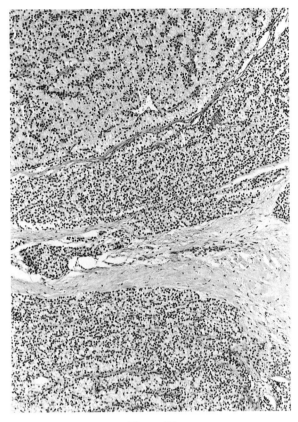

Figure 87
TERTIARY HYPERPARATHYROIDISM
ASSOCIATED WITH CHIEF CELL HYPERPLASIA
This gland shows irregular areas of fibrosis.

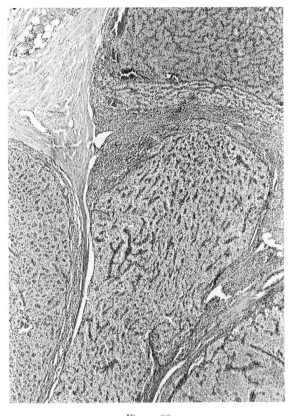

Figure 88
TERTIARY HYPERPARATHYROIDISM
ASSOCIATED WITH CHIEF CELL HYPERPLASIA
This gland shows a multinodular arrangement of prolif-
erating chief cells.

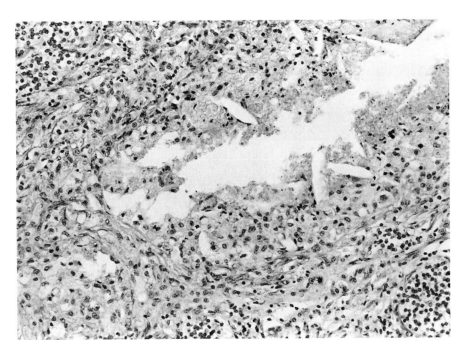

Figure 89
TERTIARY
HYPERPARATHYROIDISM
ASSOCIATED WITH
CHIEF CELL
HYPERPLASIA
A few areas of necrosis are
present in this gland.

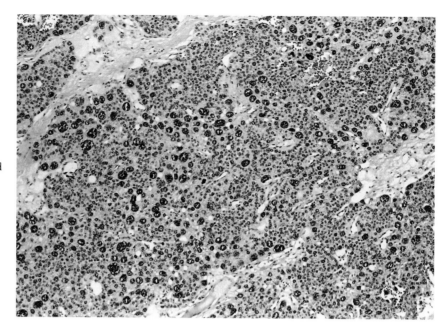

Figure 90
TERTIARY
HYPERPARATHYROIDISM
ASSOCIATED WITH
ADENOMA
Cells in this gland have enlarged
hyperchromatic nuclei.

REFERENCES

1. Akerström G, Malmaeus J, Grimelius L, Ljunghall S, Bergström R. Histological changes in parathyroid glands in subclinical and clinical renal disease. An autopsy investigation. Scand J Urol Nephrol 1984;18:75–84.

2. Altenähr E, Arps H, Montz R, Dorn G. Quantitative ultrastructural and radioimmunologic assessment of parathyroid gland activity in primary hyperparathyroidism. Lab Invest 1979;41:303–12.

3. Banerjee SS, Faragher B, Haselton PS. Nuclear diameter in parathyroid disease. J Clin Pathol 1983;36:143–8.

4. Breslau NA. Update on secondary forms of hyperparathyroidism. Am J Med Sci 1987;294:120–31.

5. Castleman B, Mallory TB. Parathyroid hyperplasia in chronic renal insufficiency. Am J Pathol 1937;13:553–74.

6. _____, Roth SI. Tumors of the parathyroid glands. Atlas of Tumor Pathology, 2nd Series, Fascicle 14. Washington, D.C.: Armed Forces Institute of Pathology, 1978:1–94.

7. Fitko R, Roth SI, Hines JR, Roxe DM, Cahill E. Parathyromatosis in hyperparathyroidism. Hum Pathol 1990;21:234–7.

8. Harlow S, Roth SI, Bauer K, Marshall RB. Flow cytometric DNA analysis of nominal and pathological parathyroid glands. Mod Pathol 1991;4:310–5.

9 Hasleton PS, Ali HH. The parathyroid in chronic renal failure—a light and electron microscopical study. J Pathol 1980;132:307–23.

10. Klempa I, Frei U, Röttger P, Schneider M, Koch KM. Parathyroid autografts—morphology and function: six years' experience with parathyroid autotransplantation in uremic patients. World J Surg 1984;8:540–6.

11. Krause MW, Hedinger CE. Pathologic study of parathyroid glands in tertiary hyperparathyroidism. Hum Pathol 1985;16:772–84.

12. Pappenheimer AM, Wilens SL. Enlargement of the parathyroid glands in renal disease. Am J Path 1935;11:73–91.

13. Roth SI, Marshall RB. Pathology and ultrastructure of the human parathyroid glands in chronic renal failure. Arch Intern Med 1969;124:397–407.

14. Salusky IB, Coburn JW. The renal osteodystrophies. In: DeGroot LJ, ed. Endocrinology, Vol 2. 2nd ed. Philadelphia: WB Saunders, 1989:1032.

15. San-Juan J, Monteagudo C, Fraker D, Norton J, Merino MJ. Significance of mitotic activity and other morphologic parameters in parathyroid adenomas and their correlation with clinical behavior [Abstract]. Am J Clin Pathol 1989;92:523.

16. Sitges-Serra A, Caralps-Riera A. Hyperparathyroidism associated with renal disease. Pathogenesis, natural history and surgical treatment. Surg Clin North Am 1987;67:359–77.

17. Snover DC, Foucar K. Mitotic activity in benign parathyroid disease. Am J Clin Pathol 1981;75:345–7.

18. St Goar WT. Case records of the Massachusetts General Hospital (Case 29-1963). Castleman B, Kibbee BO, eds. N Engl J Med 1963;268:943–53.

19. Wallfelt C, Larsson R, Gylfe E, Ljunghall S, Rastad J, Akerström G. Secretory disturbance in hyperplastic parathyroid nodules of uremic hyperparathyroidism—implication for parathyroid autotransplantation. World J Surg 1988;12:431–8.

20. Wells SA Jr, Ellis GJ, Gunnels JC, Schneider AB, Sherwood LM. Parathyroid autotransplantation in primary parathyroid hyperplasia. N Engl J Med 1976;295:57–62.

21. _____, Gunnels JC, Shelburne JD, Schneider AB, Sherwood LM. Transplantation of the parathyroid glands in man: clinical indications and results. Surgery 1975;78:34–44.

MISCELLANEOUS LESIONS

PARATHYROID CYST

Parathyroid cysts are rare lesions that can present in the neck or mediastinum (2,4,5). Cervical parathyroid cysts are considerably more common than those occurring within the mediastinum. The most common preoperative diagnosis is cystic thyroid nodule (8). Mediastinal parathyroid cysts may also contain small fragments of thymus (9). Cysts containing both thymus and parathyroid are sometimes referred to as *third pharyngeal pouch cysts*. While some cysts develop as a result of degeneration of parathyroid adenomas or hyperplasia (1,7), others have a developmental origin (8).

Parathyroid cysts, which may measure up to 10 cm in diameter, are loosely attached to the thyroid, with a definite cleavage plane. The cyst walls are typically grey-white, translucent, paper thin, and membranous (figs. 91, 92). The cyst fluid is usually thin, watery, and straw-colored; occasionally, the cyst fluid is bloody or opalescent. Such cysts may develop as remnants of the third or fourth branchial cleft along the normal pathway of embryologic migration. Alternatively, these cysts may represent persistent Kursteiner canals which are found in association with the developing parathyroid. It has also been suggested that large parathyroid cysts may result from coalescence of microcysts (8).

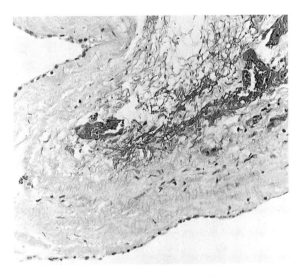
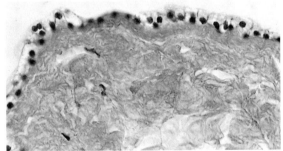

Figure 92
PARATHYROID CYST

In most areas the cyst is lined by flattened epithelial cells (top). In some areas, the lining cells have a clear cytoplasm and resemble vacuolated chief cells (bottom). There was no evidence of hyperparathyroidism.

Figure 91
PARATHYROID CYST

Intact parathyroid cyst with thickened fibrous wall. The patient did not have hyperparathyroidism. (Fig. 95 from Fascicle 14, Second Series.)

The cyst wall is typically composed of fibrous connective tissue with entrapped islands of parathyroid chief cells. An occasional cyst may be lined by a layer of chief cells (fig. 92). In those cases resulting from degeneration of an adenoma or of a hyperplastic gland, portions of abnormal parathyroid tissue may be found in the cyst wall. However, it may be impossible to identify parathyroid tissue if extensive scarring has occurred.

SECONDARY TUMORS

Secondary involvement of the parathyroids by tumor may occur through extension from adjacent structures (thyroid, larynx) or by metastatic spread. In a prospective series of 160 autopsies of patients with cancer, Horwitz and co-workers (6) found metastasis to at least one parathyroid gland in 19 cases (11.9 percent). The most common sites of origin, in order of decreasing frequency, were breast, blood (leukemia), skin (melanoma), lung, and soft tissue. De la Monte and associates (3) described parathyroid metastases in 6 percent of patients with widely disseminated breast cancer. Hypoparathyroidism, occurring as a result of tumorous destruction of the parathyroids, however, is a rare event (3). Hypocalcemia and hyperphosphatemia were recorded in only 2 of 19 patients from the series of Horwitz (6). In both instances, more than 70 percent of the parathyroid parenchyma was replaced by tumor.

REFERENCES

1. Calandra DB, Shah KH, Prinz RA, et al. Parathyroid cysts: a report of 11 cases including two associated with hyperparathyroid crisis. Surgery 1983;94:887–92.
2. Castleman B, Roth SI. Tumors of the parathyroid glands. Atlas of Tumor Pathology, 2nd Series, Fascicle 14. Washington, D.C.: Armed Forces Institute of Pathology, 1978, 1–94.
3. de la Monte SM, Hutchins GM, Moore GW. Endocrine organ metastases from breast carcinoma. Am J Pathol 1984;114:131–6.
4. Haid SP, Method HL, Beal JM. Parathyroid cysts. Report of two cases and a review of the literature. Arch Surg 1967;94:421–6.
5. Hoehn JG, Beahrs OH, Woolner LB. Unusual surgical lesions of the parathyroid gland. Am J Surg 1969;118:770–8.
6. Horwitz CA, Myers WP, Foote FW Jr. Secondary malignant tumors of the parathyroid glands. Report of two cases with associated hypoparathyroidism. Am J Med 1972;52:797–808.
7. Shields TW, Staley CJ. Functioning parathyroid cysts. Arch Surg 1961;82:937–42.
8. Wang C, Vickery AL Jr, Maloof F. Large parathyroid cysts mimicking thyroid nodules. Ann Surg 1972;175:448–53.
9. Wick MR. Mediastinal cysts and intrathoracic thyroid tumors. Semin Diagn Pathol 1990;7:285–94.

✧ ✧ ✧

PROCEDURES FOR PATHOLOGIC EXAMINATION

The optimal treatment of patients with hyperparathyroidism requires a close working relationship between the pathologist, endocrinologist, and surgeon (5–7). The pathologist should be apprised of any pertinent history relating to previous endocrine disorders and the family history. Ideally, the pathologist should be present in the operating room to observe the exposed parathyroid glands in situ. If this is not possible, the pathologist should at least know whether the biopsy is from a normal sized or enlarged gland. Depending on variations in the distribution of chief cells in a parathyroid gland and on constitutional factors, biopsy of a normal sized gland may appear hypercellular and the pathologist might erroneously make a diagnosis of hyperplasia. On the other hand, biopsy of a hyperplastic gland or adenoma containing abundant stromal fat might be misinterpreted as a normal gland without knowledge of the gland size (1).

INTRAOPERATIVE AND FROZEN SECTION EXAMINATION

Upon receipt by the pathologist, each intact gland or biopsy specimen should first be labeled as to anatomic site. Each specimen should be measured and weighed after removing the surrounding fat but before sampling for frozen section examination. The gross description should include information on the external appearance, color, and consistency of each gland. At the time of frozen section, additional sections should be retained for examination with fat stains, as discussed below. Representative samples, if sufficient tissue is available, should also be frozen at -70°C for possible molecular studies.

The role of the pathologist during parathyroid exploration is first, to determine if the biopsied tissue is of parathyroid origin and second, to determine the nature of the underlying process (hyperplasia versus adenoma) (2,3,6).

Parathyroid may be difficult to distinguish grossly from a variety of other tissues in the neck including fat, lymph node, thyroid, and ectopic thymus. The surgeon, depending on experience, may request frozen sections on a number of such samples to confirm the presence or absence of parathyroid tissue.

Generally, the distinction between parathyroid and nonparathyroid tissue is easily accomplished by frozen section. Occasionally, however, it is difficult to differentiate a lobule of thyroid from parathyroid, particularly if the parathyroid biopsy shows follicular structures. Generally, the follicles in parathyroid tissue are smaller than those in normal thyroid and the cells have a clear or vacuolated cytoplasm. Deeper sections of such equivocal cases may reveal areas more typical of parathyroid tissue. The distinction between a fragment of microfollicular thyroid adenoma and parathyroid may be impossible on frozen section and may occasionally present considerable difficulties on permanent sections.

Fragments of ectopic thymus may be composed almost exclusively of epithelial elements that are difficult to differentiate from parathyroid. The identification of Hassal corpuscles clearly establishes a thymic origin in such instances.

Geelhoed and Silverberg (4) advocate the use of intraoperative imprints for the rapid identification of parathyroid tissue. This procedure permits cytologic evaluation in less than one minute per specimen, with accurate and reproducible determination of the presence or absence of parathyroid tissue. Pathologic diagnoses are possible on abnormal parathyroid glands when the imprint is used as a screening procedure to select specimens for subsequent frozen section examination.

The critical issue in distinguishing hyperplasia from adenoma at surgery is the determination of the number of enlarged parathyroid glands. The vast majority of patients with parathyroid adenoma will have involvement of one gland, and the remaining glands will be of normal size.

In most instances, the surgeon will remove the largest gland first. The gland should be carefully weighed and a representative section, which includes the capsule, should be selected for frozen section examination. Since a rim of adjacent parathyroid is seen in 30 to 50 percent of cases at the time of frozen section, the pathologist cannot rely on this criterion alone to render a diagnosis of adenoma (6).

The presence of stromal fat cannot be used to exclude the diagnosis of adenoma, since adenomas may contain at least some stromal fat, and some adenomas contain an abundance of stromal fat (1). In many instances, the pathologist can only report that the resected gland is hypercellular and that it may represent adenoma or hyperplasia. The surgeon must then sample another gland. If this gland is of normal size and cellularity, both the surgeon and pathologist can be satisfied that the diagnosis is most likely adenoma (5).

The diagnosis of hyperplasia is likely when more than one gland is enlarged. It should be remembered, however, that hyperplasia may not involve all glands equally and that one dominant gland may be present. Biopsy of a second gland in this situation, particularly if the biopsy is from one of the poles, may reveal a relatively high proportion of stromal fat. In such instances, it is imperative to know the size of the gland. If the second gland is enlarged, the likelihood of hyperplasia is high. Fat stains, as discussed below, are helpful in making this distinction.

PREPARATION OF TISSUES FOR PERMANENT SECTIONS

After frozen section examination, the remaining portion of each sample is fixed in formalin for the preparation of permanent sections, which are stained routinely with hematoxylin and eosin. In our laboratory, each biopsy specimen measuring less than 5 mm in diameter is sectioned at three levels. Samples measuring more than 5 mm are bisected, and each half is submitted for histologic examination.

Enlarged parathyroid glands are bisected and each half, including the capsule, is submitted for histologic examination. The thickness of the blocks should not exceed 3 mm in order to insure optimal fixation and processing. An average of two blocks per cm^3 of tissue is generally adequate.

Sections of thymic fat are generally blocked in their entirety. We have seen extensive parathyromatosis within grossly normal thymic tissue.

The final report should include the diagnosis together with the precise locations of all biopsies in order to facilitate localizing parathyroid remnants should re-exploration be necessary.

FAT STAINS

The use of fat stains for the evaluation of the parathyroids is based on the observation that the intracellular or parenchymal lipid content is decreased or absent in hyperfunctioning chief cells as compared to normal or suppressed chief cells (see pl. VIII). Some studies have stressed that evaluation of intracellular fat content is considerably more important than the estimation of stromal fat content.

Roth and Gallagher (14) employed Sudan IV stains to evaluate frozen sections of parathyroid tissue and demonstrated prominent intracellular sudanophilic deposits in up to 80 percent of chief cells of suppressed parathyroid glands. Cases of chief cell hyperplasia and adenoma, on the other hand, contained little or no stainable lipid. Similar results were obtained with oil red O.

Some authors, however, noted considerable variation in the parenchymal lipid content of hyperplasia and adenoma cases (9–12). Dufour and Durkowski (9) reported positive staining in at least one gland from patients with hyperplasia, and in five of six cases the staining was intense. Moreover, variation in intracellular fat content was seen within individual glands. Bondeson and co-workers (8) also studied the fat content of hyperplastic glands and reported considerable variation in staining in the same gland and in different glands from the same patient (see pl. IX–B). However, all hyperplastic glands showed distinctly divergent areas of parenchyma with marked reduction or absence of parenchymal fat in some foci. In 73 patients with normal glands obtained at autopsy, 15 percent had reduced sudanophilic staining, suggesting the presence of hyperfunctioning parathyroid tissue.

Monchik and co-workers (13) noted that both oil red O and Sudan IV may produce divergent results on the same specimen. They hypothesized that the organic solvents in which these dyes are dissolved may lyse or leach lipid from the tissues. Accordingly, they employed osmium-alum carmine for evaluation of parathyroid parenchymal cell fat content. The sections were first cut in a cryostat, fixed in 10 percent neutral buffered formalin, and further fixed and stained with 1 percent osmium tetroxide followed by counterstaining with alum carmine. This procedure has provided reproducible results in initial studies.

Bondeson et al. (8) examined the parathyroid glands from almost 200 cases of surgically treated hyperparathyroidism using a modified oil red O technique. On the basis of careful histologic examination and clinical follow-up, they concluded that access to two complete glands and the use of fat stains allows highly reproducible and reliable distinction between adenoma and hyperplasia. The rate of equivocal findings for cases in which two glands were available was 8 percent. As with other special procedures, fat stains should not be used alone for evaluation of parathyroid disease. However, a combination of fat stains and careful morphologic assessment provides an optimal approach.

DENSITY GRADIENTS

Density measurements provide an objective evaluation of the ratio of parenchymal to fat cells (15,16). This approach is based on the differences in density between the parenchymal cells and stromal fat cells. The medium used for density gradient measurements is Percoll equilibrated with sodium chloride to iso-osmotic conditions.

Akerström and co-workers (15) found that the density of parathyroid glands is related linearly to the parenchymal cell content. The density of the parathyroid indirectly allows an estimate of the parenchymal content, and with knowledge of the total glandular weight, it is possible to calculate the parenchymal weight.

DNA CYTOMETRY

Both static and flow cytometric methods have been used for the assessment of DNA content of proliferative lesions of the parathyroid glands (26). Most of the data now available are based on studies employing formalin-fixed, paraffin-embedded samples processed according to the method of Hedley and associates (20).

Most published studies have reported that the majority of normal parathyroids have a diploid DNA pattern (19). Some normal glands, however, exhibit small tetraploid peaks.

Studies by Irwin and co-workers (21) indicate that approximately 80 percent of adenomas contain tetraploid peaks. Other studies, however, report that this high frequency of tetraploidy may be related to the contamination of the preparations by cell aggregates. Harlow and co-workers (19) found that only 1 of 12 adenoma cases (8 percent) contained a tetraploid population. In the study of Bowlby and associates (18), 12 of 56 (21 percent) adenomas contained tetraploid populations. They found diploid DNA patterns with less than 15 percent tetraploid cells in 2 of 10 (20 percent) cases of primary chief cell hyperplasia but in no cases of secondary hyperplasia.

The frequency of aneuploidy in adenomas ranges from 3 to 25 percent in different series utilizing flow cytometry of formalin-fixed and paraffin-embedded samples (17,19,23–27). A comparable frequency of aneuploidy has been noted in parathyroid carcinomas using similar technical approaches. These findings indicate that flow cytometry is generally not a useful approach in distinguishing parathyroid adenoma from carcinoma. Moreover, aneuploidy has been reported in 20 percent of hyperplastic parathyroids from patients with secondary hyperparathyroidism (20).

Obara and co-workers (27) reported that the analysis of DNA content might be useful for the prediction of clinical outcome of patients with parathyroid carcinoma. In their study, patients with aneuploid carcinomas were more likely to have an aggressive form of the disease than those with diploid carcinomas.

Levin and co-workers (24) utilized Feulgen-stained sections to determine the DNA content of a series of benign and malignant parathyroid tumors. The mean DNA content of the carcinomas was significantly greater than that of the adenomas. Using this approach, Levin et al. found an aneuploid pattern in four of nine carcinomas but in none of the parathyroid adenomas.

Kinetic analyses of normal parathyroids show mean S-phase fractions of 1.2 percent, while mean S-phase fractions of adenomas and secondary hyperplasias are 1.5 percent and 0.8 percent, respectively (19). Carcinomas have a mean S-phase fraction of 6 percent. On the basis of these studies, Harlow and co-workers concluded that a diagnosis of carcinoma should be considered in the presence of an S-phase fraction of greater than 4 percent and a DNA index greater than 1.2.

FINE-NEEDLE ASPIRATION BIOPSY

There are relatively few studies on the use of fine-needle aspiration biopsy for the diagnosis of parathyroid proliferative lesions (30–37).

Several groups have used needle aspirates in conjunction with noninvasive preoperative procedures, including ultrasonography, thallium technetium scanning, MRI, and CT scanning. Approximately 75 percent of parathyroid neoplasms measuring more than 1 cm in diameter could be localized with this approach, including examples of mediastinal adenomas. The success rate of these procedures, however, is considerably less in patients with multiglandular disease.

Mincione and co-workers (34) reported their experience with Papanicolaou-stained aspiration biopsies in seven cases of adenomas in which the specimens were obtained under echographic control. The specimens presented a highly cellular appearance with numerous dissociated epithelial cells, as well as variably sized epithelial aggregates. The nuclei were variable in size, round to ovoid, and hyperchromatic. Numerous "naked" nuclei were evident and the chromatin was arranged in coarse granules. Nucleoli were multiple, rounded, and sometimes enlarged. The cytoplasm was pale, amphophilic, and occasionally vacuolated with ill-defined cell borders. Oncocytic cells were characterized by the presence of a more granular cytoplasm.

Davey and co-workers (30) studied clinical parathyroid aspirates from three patients as well as 15 needle aspirations or touch preparations obtained from surgical specimens. Most nuclei of adenomas measured 6 to 8 μm in diameter with occasional nuclei measuring up to 30 μm. There were no cytologic criteria to distinguish cases of hyperplasia from adenoma.

The differentiation of thyroid epithelium from parathyroid chief cells in aspirated material may be particularly difficult (31,36). In parathyroid aspirates, cell groups are thick, cohesive, and branching with frayed edges (30). Macrofollicular adenomas or adenomatous goiters have more evenly spaced "honeycomb" sheets. Aspirates from parathyroid adenomas may have a microfollicular pattern impossible to distinguish from thyroid microfollicular adenomas. While parathyroid nuclei have densely granular chromatin, the chromatin structure in thyroid follicular epithelium is often finely granular.

A colloid-like material has been seen in parathyroid aspirates. This material stains blue-green with the Papanicolaou stain, except for central regions which are more eosinophilic. Congo red–stained smears of parathyroid aspirates may reveal green birefringence within the colloid, as noted in histologic sections.

Special staining techniques have also been used to differentiate aspirated thyroid follicular cells and chief cells. Winkler and associates (37) used an immunoperoxidase technique for the localization of parathyroid hormone in aspirates, while Rastad and co-workers (35) employed the Sevier-Munger argyrophil stain for positive identification of chief cells. The number of silver-positive granules showed considerable variation between the cells of each parathyroid aspirate, although some positive cells were invariably found. Macrophages exhibited some degree of argyrophilia with the Sevier-Munger and Grimelius methods, but follicular cells were generally negative.

Fine-needle aspiration biopsies are of value when used in conjunction with CT and ultrasound imaging procedures for the identification of hyperfunctioning tissue in patients who remain hypercalcemic following surgery for hyperparathyroidism (32). Parathyroid carcinomas, in the few cases studied by this approach, have a high nuclear-cytoplasmic ratio with coarsely clumped chromatin and prominent nucleoli.

REFERENCES

Intraoperative and Frozen Section Examination

1. Abul-Haj SK, Conklin H, Hewitt WC. Functioning lipoadenoma of the parathyroid gland: report of a unique case. N Engl J Med 1962;266:121–3.
2. Akerström G, Bergström R, Grimelius L, et al. Relation between changes in clinical and histopathological features of primary hyperparathyroidism. World J Surg 1986;10:696–702.
3. Castleman R, Roth SI. Tumors of the parathyroid glands. Atlas of Tumor Pathology, 2nd Series, Fascicle 14. Washington, D.C.: Armed Forces Institute of Pathology, 1978: 1–94.
4. Geelhoed GW, Silverberg SG. Intraoperative imprints for the identification of parathyroid tissue. Surgery 1984;96:1124–31.
5. Norton JA, Aurbach GD, Marx SJ, Doppman JL. Surgical management of hyperparathyroidism. In: DeGroot LJ, ed. Endocrinology, Vol 2. 2nd ed. Philadelphia: WB Saunders, 1989: 1013–31.
6. Roth SI. The parathyroid gland. In: Silverberg SG, ed. Principles and practice of surgical pathology, Vol 2. 2nd ed. New York: Churchill-Livingstone, 1990:1923–55.
7. _____, Wang CA, Potts JT Jr. The team approach to primary hyperparathyroidism. Hum Pathol 1975;6:645–8.

Fat Stains

8. Bondeson AG, Bondeson L, Ljungberg O, Tibblin S. Fat staining in parathyroid disease—diagnostic value and impact on surgical strategy: clinicopathologic analysis of 191 cases. Hum Pathol 1985;16:1255–63.
9. Dufour DR, Durkowski C. Sudan IV stain. Its limitations in evaluating parathyroid functional status. Arch Pathol Lab Med 1982;106:224–7.
10. Kasdon EJ, Rosen S, Cohen RB, Silen W. Surgical pathology of hyperparathyroidism. Usefulness of fat stain and problems in interpretation. Am J Surg Pathol 1981;5:381–4.
11. King DT, Hirose FM. Chief cell intracytoplasmic fat used to evaluate parathyroid disease in frozen section. Arch Pathol Lab Med 1979;103:609–12.
12. Ljungberg O, Tibblin S. Preoperative fat staining of frozen sections in primary hyperparathyroidism. Am J Pathol 1979;95:633–41.
13. Monchik JM, Farrugia R, Teplitz C, Teplitz J, Brown S. Parathyroid surgery: the role of chief cell intracellular fat staining with osmium carmine in the intraoperative management of patients with primary hyperparathyroidism. Surgery 1983;94:877–86.
14. Roth SI, Gallagher MJ. The rapid identification of "normal" parathyroid glands by the presence of intracellular fat. Am J Pathol 1976;84:521–8.

Density Gradients

15. Akerström G, Grimelius L, Johansson H, Pertoft H, Lundqvist H. Estimation of the parathyroid parenchymal cell mass by density gradients. Am J Pathol 1980;99:685–94.
16. Wang C, Reider SV. A density test for the intraoperative differentiation of parathyroid hyperplasia from neoplasia. Ann Surg 1978;187:63–7.

DNA Cytometry

17. Bengtsson A, Grimelius L, Johansson H, Pontén J. Nuclear DNA-content of parathyroid cells in adenomas, hyperplastic and normal glands. Acta Pathol Microbiol Immunol Scand [A] 1977;85:455–60.
18. Bowlby L, DeBault LE, Abraham S. Flow cytometric DNA analysis of parathyroid glands. Relationship between nuclear DNA and pathologic classifications. Am J Pathol 1987;128:338–44.
19. Harlow S, Roth SI, Bauer K, Marshall RB. Flow cytometric analysis of normal and pathologic parathyroid glands. Mod Pathol 1991;4:310–5.
20. Hedley DW, Friedlander ML, Taylor IW, Rugg CA, Musgrove EA. Method for analysis of cellular DNA content of paraffin-embedded pathological material using flow cytometry. J Histochem Cytochem 1983;31:1333–5.
21. Irvin GL III, Bagwell CB. Identification of histologically undetectable parathyroid hyperplasia by flow cytometry. Am J Surg 1979;138:567–71.
22. _____, Taupier MA, Block NL, Reiss E. DNA patterns in parathyroid disease predict postoperative hormone secretion. Surgery 1988;104:1115–20.
23. Joensuu H, Klemi PJ. DNA aneuploidy in adenomas of endocrine organs. Am J Pathol 1988;132:145–51.
24. Levin KE, Chew KL, Ljung BM, Mayall BH, Siperstein AE, Clark OH. Deoxyribonucleic acid cytometry helps identify parathyroid carcinomas. J Clin Endocrinol Metab 1988;67:779–84.
25. Levin KE, Galante M, Clark OH. Parathyroid carcinoma versus parathyroid adenoma in patients with profound hypercalcemia. Surgery 1987;101:649–60.

26. Mallette LE. DNA quantitation in the study of parathyroid lesions. A review. Am J Clin Pathol 1992;98:305–11.
27. Obara T, Fujimoto Y, Hirayama A, et al. Flow cytometric DNA analysis of parathyroid tumors with special reference to its diagnostic and prognostic value in parathyroid carcinoma. Cancer 1990;65:1789–93.
28. Rosen IB, Musclow CE. DNA histogram of parathyroid tissue in determining extent of parathyroidectomy. Surgery 1985;98:1024–30.
29. Shenton BK, Ellis H, Johnston ID, Farndon JR. DNA analysis and parathyroid pathology. World J Surg 1990;14:296–301.

Fine-Needle Aspiration Biopsy

30. Davey DD, Glant MD, Berger EK. Parathyroid cytopathology. Diagn Cytopathol 1986;2:76–80.
31 Friedman M, Shimaoka K, Lopez CA, Shedd DP. Parathyroid adenoma diagnosed as papillary carcinoma of the thyroid on needle aspiration smears. Acta Cytol 1983;27:337–40.
32. Gooding GA, Clark OH, Stark DD, Moss AA, Montgomery CK. Parathyroid aspiration biopsy under ultrasound guidance in the postoperative hyperparathyroid patient. Radiology 1985;155:193–6.
33. Löwhagen T, Sprenger E. Cytologic presentation of thyroid tumors in aspiration biopsy smears: a review of sixty cases. Acta Cytol 1974;18:192–7.
34. Mincione GP, Borrelli D, Cicchi P, Ipponi PL, Fiorini A. Fine needle aspiration cytology of parathyroid adenoma. A review of seven cases. Acta Cytol 1986;30:65–9.
35. Rastad J, Johansson H, Lindgren PG, Ljunghall S, Stenkvist B, Akerström G. Ultrasonic localization and cytologic identification of parathyroid tumors. World J Surg 1984;8:501–8.
36. Sahin A, Robinson RA. Papillae formation in parathyroid adenoma. A source of possible diagnostic error. Arch Pathol Lab Med 1988;112: 99–100.
37. Winkler B, Gooding GA, Montgomery CK, Clark OH, Arnaud C. Immunoperoxidase confirmation of parathyroid origin of ultrasound-guided fine needle aspirates of the parathyroid glands. Acta Cytol 1987;31:40–4.

✧✧✧

---

* Page numbers in boldface indicate table and figure pages

✧✧✧